DRAGONTIME

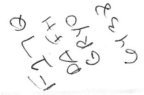

DRAGONTIME
Magic and Mystery
of Menstruation

Luisa Francia

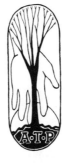

Ash Tree Publishing
Woodstock, New York

All information in *Dragontime* is based on the experiences and research of the author and other professionals. This information is shared with the understanding that you accept complete responsibility for your own health and well-being. You have a unique body and the action of each herbal medicine is unique and health care is full of variables. The result of any treatment suggested herein cannot always be anticipated and never guaranteed. The author and publisher are not responsible for any adverse effects or consequences resulting from the use of any remedies, procedures, or preparations included in this book. Consult your inner guidance, knowledgeable friends, and trained healers in addition to the words written here.

Original title: *Drachenzeit* © 1988 Luisa Francia.

English translation by Sasha Daucus.

© 1991 by Ash Tree Publishing
        PO Box 64, Woodstock, NY 12498.

Photographs except pages 138-139 © by Ine Guckert.

Illustrations on pages 34, 78, 82-95, 130 © by Mau Blossom.

Illustrations on pages 13, 19, 58, 110, 113, 121, 141 © by Alan McKnight.

Illustrations on pages 16, 22 © by Martha McGehee.

Illustrations on pages 9, 10, 11, 27, 38, 60, 61, 70, 71, 76, 77 ©by Susun Weed.

Cover art and spots except pages 40, 126 © by Susun Weed.

Library of Congress Catalog Card Number: 90-83456

ISBN 0-9614620-3-5

Printed and bound by Bookcrafters, Chelsea, Michigan, United States of America.

Printed on RECYCLED PAPER.

recycled

Table of Contents

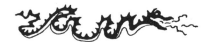

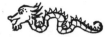

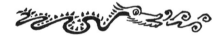

Acknowledgments

Lots of dragon-treasure smiles to:
- Sasha Daucus for a terrific translation.
- Mau Blossom, Alan McKnight, Martha McGehee, and Susun Weed for their delightful drawings.
- Ine Gunkert for her potent photographs.
- Kent Babcock for timely typesetting.
- Betsy Sandlin for picky proofreading.
- Ann Drucker and Susun Weed for exacting indexing.
- Peg Goddard for a perfect paste-up. ("Done with my own menstrual blood," she called to say.)
- The 1990 apprentices at the Wise Woman Center for ongoing support: Marji Ackerman, Regina Baskau, Cindy Belew, Chris Boardman, Annemarie Carangelo, Chris Dahl, Irmela Dehnert, Ann Drucker, Kimberly Eve, Gardenia Gardener, Regina Golding, Nora Jamieson, Kristen Johnson, Kim Lemmon, Caro Meurer, Mo O'Brien, Bärbl Pfleiderer, Alexa Petrenko, Marie Summerwood, and Ellen Weinstock.
- Kris Jeter and Robert Masters for reams of really good references.
- Brooke Medicine Eagle, Spider, Cornwoman, and Viki Noble for their moon-time inspirations.
- The women of Frauenoffensive Verlag.
- And, the sweet bloody wombs of all our mothers and grandmothers for bringing us here.

Translator's Foreword

During the months that I worked on translating *Dragontime*, I found myself immersed in a strange and wondrous world. The landscape of *Dragontime* is one populated with fire-breathing dragons, witches, and pot-bellied cauldrons; filled with caves, glowing softly red, and ice-gray mountain crags. A landscape of round hills, like pregnant bellies, crisscrossed by roads leading deeper into a land of myth, truth, and self-discovery. One sound kept me company, the sound of blood, dripping, flowing, dissolving, and nourishing.

In another reality, my everyday life, I'm a midwife and woman's health care practitioner. Everyday I see women who in some way or another are dealing in very real ways with blood, their blood. Some of these women are nourishing a baby with their blood. Others want their blood to flow, but with less pain, or more often, or not quite as much. Still others are moving into menopause and want to understand and nurture this change in their cycle. As I worked on the book, these women were with me and gave me inspiration.

Dragontime is a book with the power to heal, to transmute pain into growth, expansion, and health. Because it's more than a book of fantasy creatures. Luisa's dragons come from our own dreams and "inner mythology." Her mythical world rings true in ways that "facts" will never achieve. As a translator, I have tried to preserve the unique integrity of this evocative world, where the sound of our own woman's blood is the clue leading us back to ourselves and to our own inner power.

Sasha Daucus
Doniphan, Missouri
September, 1990

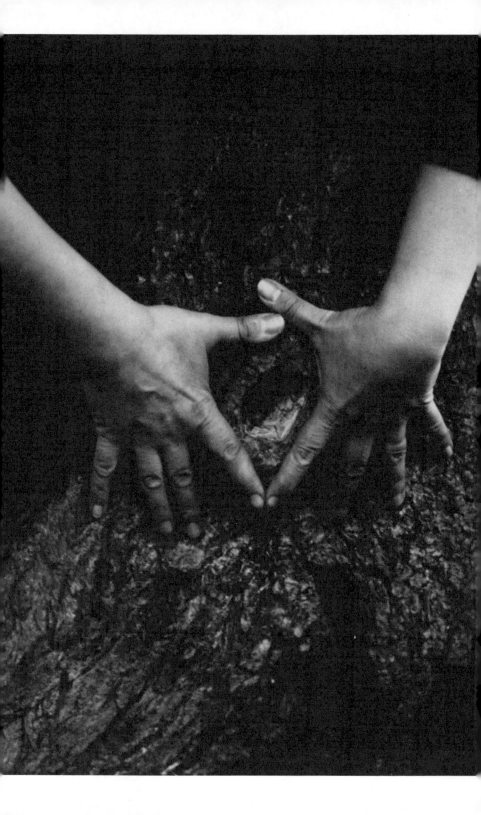

Introduction

When I went seeking vision on the sacred mountain of my ancestors, Bear Butte, a line of ancient Grandmother spirits danced around me, and I was given a very strong message for women by one called Rainbow Woman, Woman of Rainbow Light. She spoke to me of our responsibility as women, of the charge we accept and carry as we choose to come into a female body for our Earthwalk. She instructed us, "As an Earth woman, you carry the responsibility for the nurturing and renewing of all life. The Great Mystery creates human life through your womb and gives you breasts to nurture your children. This understanding given you in your bodies must be modeled and taught to all others, so that *all* the children of All Our Relations in the entire circle of life are nurtured and renewed through the *feminine* in each person, both male and female."

She reminded me that this does not mean that women must actually *do* all the nurturing and renewing of life, but must model and teach it so clearly that all others may gain that way of being within themselves. As well, she reminded me of the primary influence of mothers on both boys and girls: through gentle, bonding birthing practices; which influence continues after birth through the precious months we hold and care for these infants, as their brains and nervous systems develop; and on through all the ways we teach them in their childhood.

So, we as women have a big job on our hands: as the crucial issues we face on Earth can also be resolved by the teachings that women know best—to nurture and renew life in all its forms—to be in good relationship with all things and all beings. We must find more and more ways to teach this, and to make it real to every person on Earth, so that the separation and fearfulness which lead to disharmony and destruction will cease. And we need powerful tools for this task.

We have those tools in the spiritual practice of our moon time— dragontime. As we begin to use the cycle of our bleeding in a visionary way, we have the most powerful tool on Earth for creating new ways of being and doing. No longer do women need to take on the macho, muscular, linear, masculine ways so often assumed in the early feminist days of searching for our power. We are now finding the true power of simply flowing with and being in good relationship with the great river of life—floating gently down, rather than using force to row against the current. As the moon covers her face, as we draw near our time of bleeding, the veil between us and the Great Mystery thins. We women at that time are in the most receptive form that the human (female) ever touches. And there, in that place of retreat to the quiet of the moon lodge, we have the opportunity to leave behind the outer world of work and busyness—to retreat into visionary quiet for the nurturing of our deepest selves. In this quiet questing place, we have the ability to see deep into mystery, and to draw forth from the great starry womb of the feminine the visions, ideas, discoveries, and creative sparks which need to be made real in the lives of our people. During this monthly dragontime, our native grandmothers say we must not pray for ourselves, but for All Our Relations; so that what we bring through is for the good of all. When we are not using that precious blood to bring through a human child, then we give it away in return for other gifts of creativity which we can then manifest in the more outward, active time of the full moon."

As we begin to nurture and renew ourselves, our *deepest* selves, through moon lodge visioning retreats every month, then we will resonate into our worlds the nurturing and renewal energy that is so needed upon our Mother Earth. Remembering that we each have alive within us the knowledge given by the Great Spirit, by Mother Earth, and Grandmother Moon, we will commune together, cry and dance and dance and create, as one people.

Luisa has compiled a simmering cauldron of thoughts, ideas, stories, and exercises to help you use your dragontime well. Take these things, practice them, and go forth to create a banquet for yourself and All Our Relations—to fertilize and re-green the garden of Earth with dragon magic!

Brooke Medicine Eagle
Sky Lodge, Montana
September 1990

A native way of working with the moon time is offered in Brooke's cassette teaching tapes, Moon Time *and* Moon Lodge, *available through Harmony Network, PO Box 2550, Guerneville, CA 95446, (707) 869-0989.*

DRAGONTIME
Blood Mysteries

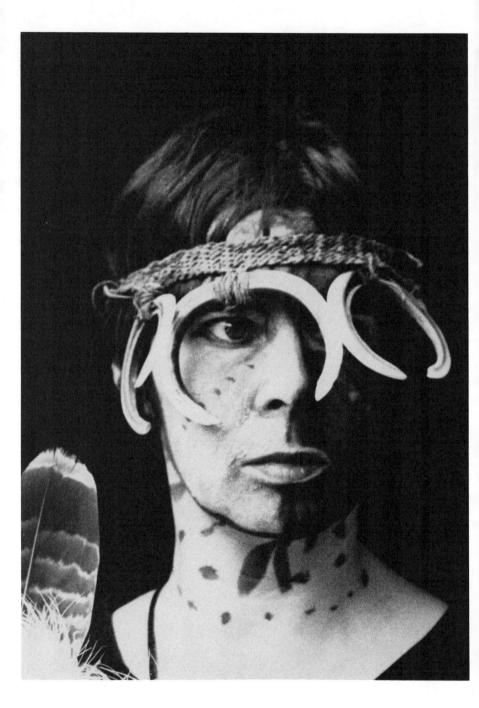

Blood Mysteries:
Tracing Down the Myths
of Menstruation

I'm sitting on the ceremonial grounds of an old Dogon village in Mali. The Dogon, still around today, live in a new village. As time has passed, they've nearly all converted to Islam. In the old village here there's only one very old woman and two old men who remain to stay in contact with the ancient ones. They're supplied with food by the women of the other village. They do not go into the new village.

But when the women of the new village menstruate, they return to the old houses, into the protection of the ancestral spirits. They isolate themselves from the business and bustle of the village and immerse themselves in the spirit world of the ancestors. The old village is now a sacred menstrual site.

I'm five years old. I go with my relatives to a Catholic church. I see a picture of a man brutally stabbing a dragon. I burst into tears.

I see church after church with one gruesome dragon-slaying motif after another. Blood everywhere. Jesus bleeds on the cross, the dead dragon bleeds. The only one who doesn't bleed is Maria.

I'm eight. My favorite stores are fairy tales. My favorite: *The Magic Steed*. "But as quickly as the young man hacked a head off the dragon, three more grew in its place, more horrible yet." I'd love to be able to do that, too: grow horrible heads.

The dragons of my childhood: my grandma, the house dragon. "You little dragon," says my mother when she thinks I'm smarting off, but can't help laughing.

The Tatzelserpent of Wendelstein, in the mountains where we often go hiking, excites my curiosity, just like Lindworm Street in Munich where my aunt lives, or Worm Lake. I picture a huge soft worm and see myself running off along it. My feet tickle the worm, which laughs fire.

"You and your vivid imagination," says my mother.

Once a month, an old enamel pot sits in the bathroom. Swimming in it are white rags with red stains. The water is reddish-brown. It smells. The cloth pads are soaked, washed, and then put, never quite white, still with interesting brown stains and somewhat darker edges, on a particular shelf in the bathroom. Our bathroom has no key. There are only women in our family.

I'm having *my time*, says my mother. It really is her time. At any rate, it's not ours. She's unapproachable. "You're a real dragon when you have your period," says my Grandma. "Indisposed," she says, too. To be indisposed. A strange disposition; a different time, outside of normal time/real time, *my time* or *my days* stand out, become the **period**.

My mother doesn't have any special pain, she's just impatient. She's listening to something inside herself. Far from us two daughters and Grandma, she's in another time. Dragontime. My mother is usually cheerful, sometimes angry. But when she's having her period, she's nervous, edgy, like a caged animal. She remembers something. But what? No one can figure it out. No one knows.

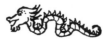

I'm sitting on the school bench, sixth grade. Something runs, warm and pleasant, out of my vagina. I know it. It's *my time*. I just take my school bag and run home. I run to my mother, in the office, and tell her. She smiles. "Don't scream like that," she says. Time of secrets. Why can't anyone hear? Don't all women have *it*? Yes, but don't *talk* about it. Men. I think of my little peeks at pregnant women. The fat belly, somehow so vulnerable. And now the blood. Vulnerable, too. We keep it to ourselves. Tell no one. We talk about it while we're eating. Grandma doesn't have *it* any more. And now I'm the last to finally get it. Every one grins. Now I belong. I'm grown up. A woman.

Men didn't stay in power long in my family. There's no place for men at the fire of the House Dragon, amidst fourfold gossip, the fire of Xanthippes and the Sphinxes. We fight and scream at each other but there's no boss in the patriarchal sense. The head of the family is the one with the most force to plow her way through. Not infrequently the youngest. Which doesn't mean there aren't any authoritarian decrees. But authority is changeable, doubted, given up, built up anew, forgotten. It's never something irrevocable. And there's never *"no more discussion on that topic."*

My mother's illogical. Her words don't add up. Nothing is final. "Don't go there anymore . . ." she says, but she lets you go again. "No time to drink cocoa . . ." then cocoa's made. "Now it's really bedtime . . ." and we sit around for hours playing dominos.

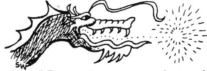

My grandma is a widow. A merry widow, say the neighbors. She has a friend, Rosie, and the two of them hop from bar to bar. We're amazed at Rosie. She is fat and crude and ancient (about 50).

Together they shake up every bar and every public dance.

My aunt rides a motorcycle and smokes 80 cigarettes a day. She has an unbelievably loud voice. (Africa's the only place I know where women, standing elbow to elbow, scream to each other as loudly as the women in our family scream.)

My mother's soft and rather shy. Much too good. We think she lets herself be used.

My sister's big and strong, just like I want to be. "But if that's what you really want, you have to eat up," that's what they say. I'm describing this family so exactly because it's a Dragon Family: dragons only have Mothers and Grandmothers, Aunts and Sisters.

I know the scaly skin of Dragontime women, hot and pleasant. The sly, sometimes mean eyes. The biting remarks, the sulphur smoking out of their mouths. The columns of fire from their bad moods, the smoke of their rages, the fires of their aggression, the tar that lays over their spirits when depressions come.

The screeching laughter of women playing cards in the kitchen was the lullaby of my childhood. With so much laughter and giggling, everything must be fine.

Frequently, the family meanders into Dragontime simultaneously.

The cramps. The heavy sensation before it begins. The tension. The feelings that stagnate until they're finally spit out with fire. We're sarcastic, ready for a fight, unforgiving, self-pitying, sentimental, tender, complaining, laughing, and moaning. Then comes the blood. Maybe a hot water bottle will help. My sister slams the bathroom door in my face because I want in. "Beat it! Can't you ever leave me alone?"

When we're all out of sorts, Grandma shakes her head over the lot of us, over all our "crap."

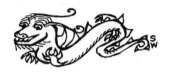

I'm thirty-six. We're camping out in an isolated valley in the Tassili mountains of the Algerian Sahara, surrounded by thousands of kilometers of sand and rock. Behind me something moves in the pitch black night. There's nothing there but a tall crag. It can't have moved. And yet, the peak bends itself down towards me. A smoldering, sulphurous light. We've set up our tent among three ancient dragons. Two of the dragons are still asleep.

Dragons want to wake.

Did someone speak?

I sit at the foot of the crags, wrapped in my sleeping bag, thinking.

Why do dragon slayers roll around in dragon blood?

Think about it.

Painted in red. Rolling in blood. The body painted with blood. Blood and power. The power of many women bleeding together . . .

It's not men who bleed, is it? The dragon's blood isn't *their* blood.

Blood is a symbol for power. Possess the symbol, you possess the power. Get the blood, you get the person's essence. Consume it, it becomes part of you. Cannibalistic peoples of Africa [and elsewhere] ate whatever part of their opponent they most feared/admired.

Blood.

Dragon blood.

Stay awake.

Think.

But I fall asleep.

And the next morning I know: I will awaken the dragons. I will tell their stories, their Dragontime tales, the blood mysteries.

Dragons in Ancient Times

We could just forget about dragons, like giants and dwarves, ghosts and fairies, or let them vegetate somewhere on the edge of our fantasies. Dragons don't *exist*, you know. Sure, there are dinosaurs. You can still admire *them* in natural history museums. But dinosaurs aren't dragons.

There are few prehistoric or preliterate depictions of dragons. Virtually every known picture or description of dragons, including flying snakes, lions with wings, fire spewing sphinxes, monsters with dragon tails, even the naming of a constellation "Draco," occurs after the development of writing.

And by the time dragons are presented in European literature and culture, the tone is moralistic—dragons are demonized, a reflection of how much they are feared.

In China, just as in Asia and South America, the dragon is a symbol of power and brings good luck.

I might never have gotten so deeply involved with dragons if the Catholic Church hadn't been so vehement about those dragon fights. There were no dragons and there are no dragons. Why then, these dragon slayings? Dragons have never been any real danger or even a remote threat of any kind. How can a religion, still practiced and taught today, take legendary dragon fights so seriously? Why these bloodthirsty depictions, this unappetizing rolling-around-in-blood?

Of course, the Catholic Church fathers had me somewhat acclimatized to holy brutality: they nail up their hero, idolize his pain, set a crown of thorns upon him; then drink his blood, eat his flesh and praise this symbolic cannibalism as holy.

So it shouldn't have amazed me that they sent out angels and saints to murder dragons. But I make it a habit to question myself when anything sticks in my head. I ask myself, "Where does this come from?" And, "Against whom is it directed?"

One ancient dragon-serpent known is *Tiamat*. Chaldean ceramics and inscriptions from 3000 B.C.E. show her as a dragon, though she could take any form. In one depiction, she stands on two animal legs and has a feathered body.

Tiamat was the Mesopotamian primeval mother. She existed in the time when "the nothing which was above was not yet named heaven, and the nothing which was below was not yet named earth." Indeed, Tiamat was the originator, creator, and birthmother of the entire universe, a woman, honored for her power to create out of her own body. From her dragon body, Tiamat birthed the earth and the waters.

Tiamat is the queen of dreams and fears. The queen of the deeps is Tiamat.

Tiamat, also known as Tohu Bohu, is Creatress of the four female elements: the night, the deeps, the water, and eternity. She is the life-giving, death-bringing dragon. Her first born child was Mummu, an image of herself.

Tiamat formed the earth from her menstrual blood, and even today, her menstrual place, the east coast of the Red Sea, is called Tihamat.

The recording of time began with menstrual calendars: marked and notched bones or small vessels containing 29 or 30 little holes and little pegs to count the days. They are said to go back to Tiamat and her menstrual blood. The earliest date back to 24,000 B.C.E.

The Babylonians honored Tiamat and the creative power of menstruation. Their hieroglyph for "woman" was a symbol literally meaning "goddess of the house." So it's not surprising that they also revered Tiamat as Creator-Mother. Before the world was created, said the Babylonians, there was only Tiamat, the dragon woman of bitter waters and sweet springs. In a timeless infinity of eternal creation, Tiamat gives birth.

Tiamat births monsters, storms, and beings which exist only in our dreams. She also bears sons and gods, and gives them homes in the far corners of the universe. But they aren't satisfied. Marduk, her son, wishes to kill her. He wants to be mightier than the Creatress, Tiamat, who bore him. Here is the primeval story: he is born of her body, born of her blood, wanting her power, wanting her blood. The son kills her and has nothing.

In the earliest versions of the myth, Marduk, the sun/son, attacks his mother Tiamat, ruler of the deep, but she merely eats him, taking him into the night of her universe to spit him out anew.

In later versions of the myth, Marduk splits Tiamat in two halves with his sword. He kills and conquers the mother and takes her power. His act of murder is declared a hero's deed and defended by renaming Tiamat "the Dragon of Chaos."

We've internalized this most ancient conquest of the primeval mother so thoroughly that some feminist lexicons don't even list Tiamat, only Marduk.

Another ancient dragon is Lilith. Adam is said to have tried to marry her, but she refused him and lifted herself up into the air, returning to her home on the Red Sea (!).

The Red Sea is "the ocean of blood that brings forth all things."

Lilith is a primeval dragon, a primeval demon, feared by all, conquered by none. She can only die "on Judgment Day." Lilith is connected with the Hebrew "Laila"—the night. It's said of her that she "did not open herself up to man . . . she did not open her clothes up in front of her man."

This is similar to descriptions of Ishtar, the "Red Goddess of Babylon," whose priestesses introduced the moon-menstrual calendars of Babylon and held initiation rites for the first menstruation and, thus, the rite of passage celebration for young girls entering into womanhood. Here, too, the *Red* Goddess is a reference to menstrual blood, just as the *Red* Sea is a reference to the primeval cauldron of all life: the womb with its menstrual blood.

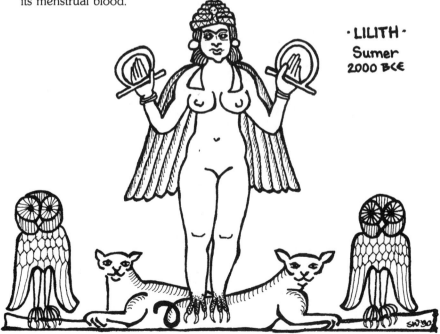

· LILITH ·
Sumer
2000 BCE

The Greek "stringes," and the "striges" of Roman mythology are the successors of Lilith and are described in *Lilith, die erste Eva* (*Lilith, the Original Eve*, Siegmund Hurwitz, 1983) thusly:

> Greedy birds are they. They fly about at night. They search out children, when their nurse is gone. They carry them away. They spoil their bodies with their claws. They are said to tear out the bowels of nurslings with their claws. Their gorge is filled with blood they drink. . . .

Gruesome dragons that eat nurslings? We're closing in on the chief anxiety of the ruling patriarchy: the bleeding woman, dependent on no one, belonging to no one, domesticated by no one, practicing her own birth control.

Here's another description of this demon, "Black Striga":

> Black Striga, black upon black.
> Blood will she eat, and blood will she drink.
> As an ox does she bellow.
> As a bear, does she roar.
> As a wolf, does she ravage.

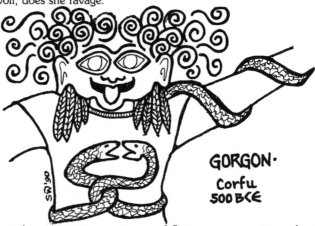

GORGON·
Corfu
500 BCE

The earliest dragons, sea monsters, and flying sea serpents are honored and named; they are goddesses who bring fertility and death. Charybdis, the sea monster, could swallow whole ships. Her friend Scylla, the sea dragon, had twelve feet, six necks, six horrible heads, and a body ending in two dolphin tails. The Unsas of Arabian myth are described without fear, indeed with a good deal of friendliness, as flying snakelike women, goddesses, who, when honored and supplicated, would give advice and assistance and who had oracular powers.

When patriarchy gains sway, the myths and stories change. Things once thought good and important become demonized. The primeval snake-mother, the goddess from whom life and death comes, is reviled and attacked. Her blood, which brought forth the earth and all its beings, is now cursed.

Now myths tell of men giving birth: Zeus for instance, who bears Athena from his head. What a metaphor of the historical situation: the time of brain children had begun. War is declared on women.

So it is that the Gorgon sisters, breathtakingly beautiful, but equally frightening in their untouchableness and freedom, evolve into disgusting, stinking creatures with snake hair and scaly bodies. They live at the end of the world, the other side of time (between the worlds of the matriarchy and the patriarchy, we could also say). Their dragon heads are covered with sulphurous scales, and on their backs they bear mighty wings.

Like many of the early primeval goddesses, the Gorgons are a triad: their names are Medusa ("wisdom"), Stheno ("strength"), and Euryale ("the wide sea"). The moon is sometimes known as the "Gorgon head."

Yet Athena, poor daughter of Zeus's head, carries a shield showing the head of Medusa. This warlike goddess, claimed by and oriented towards the masculine, thus acknowledges the power and might that she still embodies, the power and might of the woman-who-bleeds, the dragon.

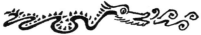

The sea dragon, Echidna, who birthed Scylla and Charybdis, is also the mother of the feared Hydra, a hideous dragon. In tales of dragon slayings and heroic campaigns against monsters, Hercules is squared off against Hydra. And though he kills her, her blood is so lethal that just one drop of it woven into his victor's cloak proves fatal to him. Here we have a first indication that a dragon's blood is a very special substance, indeed.

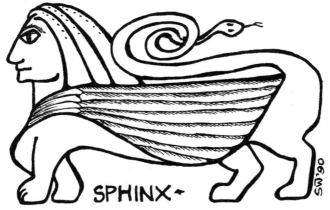

SPHINX

Another daughter of Echidna is the Sphinx, the lion woman with dragon wings. She has remained virtually untouched during the changing of the myths, for in her rests the wisdom of the wild woman and those who challenge her are destroyed.

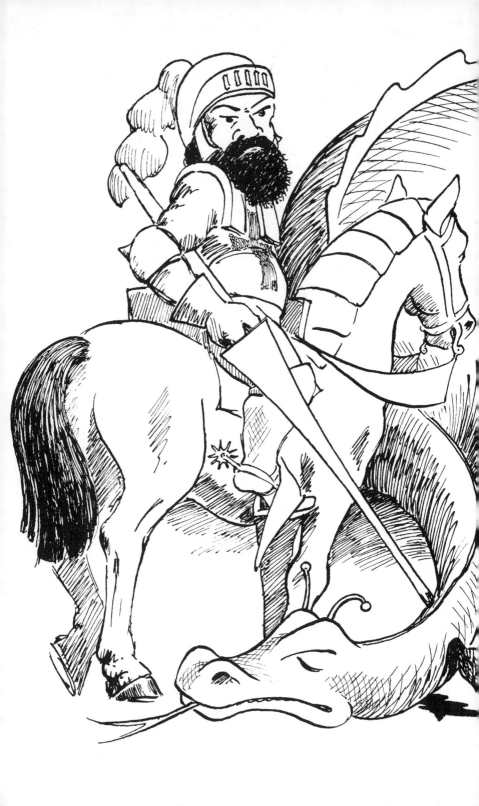

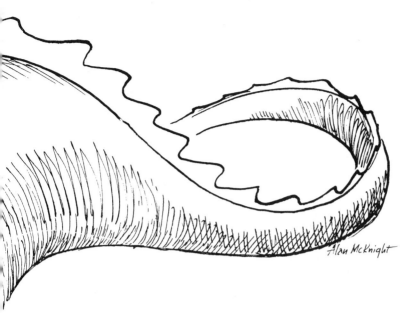

Slaying Dragons: The New Era

Dragons and their sisters are regarded with awe, honor, and reverence in early literate societies. In ancient Greece and Rome, and the even more ancient cultures of Chaldea, Sumeria, and Babylonia, dragons, as well as sea monsters, flying snakes, winged lions, and demons of the night, are respected as the dispensers of life and death.

But as patriarchal leaders, with their wrathful, solitary, male god, take power, dragons become synonymous with evil. The new male, mono-theistic hierarchies can't afford to tolerate goddess worship nor any symbols of the power of the female creative force.

The dragonly womanly might of Tiamat, Lilith, and Hydra are de-meaned. Dragontime, bleeding time, becomes taboo. And menstruating women become demons of evil, not dragons of power.

Hercules battles Hydra. Medusa is murdered unmercifully. Myths are altered in ever greater number. Words like "gruesome," "repulsive," and "terrifying" are added to descriptions of primeval goddesses. The patriarchs hope to annihilate the memory of the goddesses' powers.

Son now *must* kill Mother, for she possesses weird, dark powers. Her horrifying menstrual blood, dripping with moonlike regularity into the earth, is the seat of her power. No man can command this blood, the center of all life and death, mightiest substance of all. So the patriarchs cannot allow women this power. But they can't deny that women bleed. Instead they try to make menstrual blood their own. They reinvent it as the substance of immortality (life only, rather than mortality—life and death).

But archetypes persist.

Hercules dies from a mere drop of Hydra's blood. Does this reveal his weakness or her power?

Achilles is dipped in the River Styx (the goddess' menstrual flow, the dark river) to gain invulnerability. But something goes wrong and he's mortally wounded on the one famous spot left bare. Why isn't he really invulnerable?

Siegfried of Germanic mythology has the same trouble. He battles a dragon, kills it, and rolls around in the blood to make himself invulnerable. But, too bad for him, a leaf sticks to his shoulder, one place is left bare, and here Hagen later thrusts in his sword, killing the hero. Why?

Blood. Men kill for it, roll in it, paint themselves with it, try to make it a part of their own body, claim it as the substance of immortality. But it doesn't keep them alive. Why?

Women know these masculine heroes can't bleed the way moon-blood flows. Men's blood flows only in injury or death, with war, in slaughter and conflict. Our menstrual blood, our primeval dragontime blood, is a mighty substance, not owned by the heroes of the new era. An uncontrollable substance, a threatening power.

Then, in certain areas, the Christian Church emerges as the only acceptable spirituality of the new patriarchal order. Its dogma is not really born full-grown out of anyone's head (like Athena), but follows from the older matriarchal order and brings with it symbols and customs honoring female power and the goddess. The ancient symbols are etched into the psyches of priest and people alike: these symbols will not disappear. So their meanings must change. Like the old myths, the symbols must be made to fit in with the new philosophy. The goddess is transformed into the madonna. Angels take the place of the flying female beings, freed of their bothersome gender, neutralized. They become ethereal beings, of minor significance, and easy to deal with.

But still a female presence dominates the life of spirit and imagination. This power is still so deeply respected that amulets and charms in the shape of female sexual organs are in use everywhere, and menstrual blood talismans are used to increase strength. Eventually, the amulets, too, find a place in the new religion: the Virgin Mary is set inside a mandala which looks suspiciously like a vagina. Her blood flow is diverted, becoming sacrificial blood. With that, the transformation is complete.

From the goddess flows blood and milk, gifts of life, returning always to nourish her when those she has nourished die. All is sacred.

From the god flows blood and tears, taken from victims. Blood of Jesus: "This is my blood, which I have shed for thee." The endless return is obscured, denied. Death becomes the taking of life. Bloody sacrifice is now deemed religious. And menstrual blood, blood of peace, is declared taboo.

The new religions of wrathful monotheism establish themselves as dominant, but old beliefs, old archetypes, old goddesses live on. The dragons of old times are very powerful; they rumble around in people's heads. As people accepted the new religion and abandoned the old customs, their memories of the ancient goddess rites was a constant source of unrest. The Church had to conquer the old dragons and quiet the consciences of the flock.

Look for instance at this little rhyme from the Christian Church in which the dragon "from long ago" (not a really powerful or present force, after all) comes along and does bad things to people. (So why worship him [sic]?)

> Once long ago a dragon there was. Alleluia.
> He came and he gobbled the people all up. Alleluia.

The saints slay dragons to satisfy and comfort the people. Archangel Gabriel (one of those sexless flying beings) slays dragons; so does St. George, and St. Michael. The Church is victorious over pagan sinfulness and the uncontrollable dragon: bleeding power of women.

And what of the patriarchal "brainchildren"? The Athenas? Do these women conquer dragons too? Margaret kills the dragon with her own hands. Martha, the holy, walks the dragon on a leash. Yes, women will betray themselves, will try to confine, and rigidly control their own power and sexuality and that of other women.

The following magic spell from the Nahe Valley, Germany, said to get rid of unwanted disease, could easily be talking about what happened to the women:

> To the river, so it goes,
> Went the dragon with the rose.
> The dragon was drowned
> And the rose can't be found.

The rose is a metaphor for woman's sexuality. The blood mysteries (dragon) and women's sexuality (rose) are drowned. They vanish, leaving only a river of tears behind.

The respectable women of the Church are the mystical ones: abbesses who stifle their bodies, women with visions, heroines who sacrifice themselves and save others instead of living their own lives. Human values follow the new myths. Life and death are no longer a holy wholeness, one following from the other in endless self-renewing power, like a snake shedding her skin, like a dragon. New life—mythical, elevated, detached, pure (unreal) life—is alone worth honor.

Conscious awareness of and attention to natural fertility cycles fades. Death and menstruation become hidden, obscured, weighed down with anxiety and grief.

The Sun Hero conquers the Mother of the Night, the Moon Goddess. The Latin word *mens* meaning both "month" and "menstruation" is dropped from use. Now one lives eternally and if one does die, there's resurrection on the third day. [It's not so hard to see vestiges of the triple goddess here.]

Bless the good Therese von Konnersreuth who left a trail for me. She was accused of dripping menstrual blood from her hands and feet.

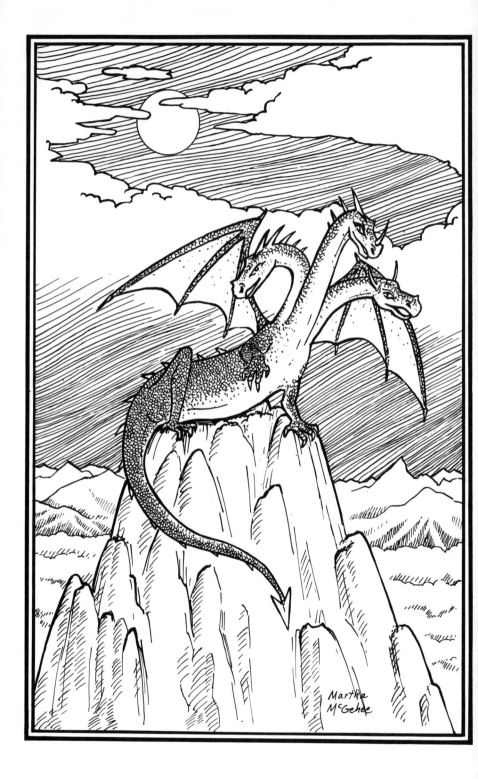

Dragon Tales

A rich vein of information about dragons can be mined in modern myths, legends, and fairy tales. Here's what I've unearthed about dragons.

Dragons have one head or many, especially seven or three. Chop off dragons' heads and they grow back again.

Dragons have grandmothers. Dragons have daughters. The fearsome dragon mother hunts down all intruders into the mythical forest.

Dragons are demanding. Dragons swallow down people and spit them out again. Dragons require a maiden every year in tithe, or they'll destroy the land. Dragons spit fire.

Princesses are watched over by dragons. The princess in the shape of a dragon lives hidden behind the blue mountains. Dragons put spells on princesses.

Heroes fight with dragons. It's not the older, stronger, brother who succeeds, but the young, innocent one. You have to serve a dragon for three or seven years.

Aid a dragon or free it from difficulty, and in return the dragon will help you and give you happiness. Wake a dragon and spare its life, and you'll be richly rewarded. Dragons can make you invulnerable.

Dragons possess nothing; their job is to guard. Dragons guard many treasures: pearls, palaces, magical forests, magical mountains, and fertile women.

Dragons live in the sea. Dragons live on mountains. Dragons appear in the shape of mist and clouds. Dragons live at the end of the world. Dragons exist on the other side of time, between heaven and earth.

Dragons are older than time. Dragons speak in the primeval language of creation. No one can gaze into a dragon's eye, for its glance is so profoundly wise and old that no mortal soul can bear its look.

Dragons are house spirits or magical beings "on the other side of time," and "between the worlds." They chiefly appear to watch over maidens and precious stones, and to protect treasures of great magical importance.

Storm and wild weather, as well as fire, are attributed to dragons and equally so to witches. Who knows if maybe they aren't one and the same. . . . Dragons are often associated with witches, who fly at night, and "step over the edge."

The dragonstone of ancient myth is often cited as being the famous carbuncle (almandite), or bloodstone, which, like all red stones, is associated with menstruation and recommended for problems of a woman's blood flow (by Hildegard von Bingen, for instance).

The close relationship between menstruation and dragons is indicated in folk tales through the fact that the same things are said of dragons and menstruating women: they crave mineral stones, everything they touch dies, and their eyes have a destructive, magical power. Their steamy breath is poisonous. their blood drops leave behind a fatal trail. (Many cultures have the superstition which warns against walking under a ladder or apple tree in case a drop of blood from a menstruating woman should fall on you.)

Dragons also appear in folk tales as grain dragons, showing their close relationship to fertility. They bring grain and with it, life, for grain is fulfillment, nourishment, the full belly, the mother, milk of the Goddess.

Rose Maiden

An orphan boy, raised by a woods-woman, experiences such a yearning for the Rose Maiden that he determines to leave his loving foster mother.

"It is far my son, and should you manage to reach her, you will still face many difficulties for she is watched over by a dragon," says the woods-woman.

But the boy will go, so she gives him a little round magic bell, saying, "If you need anything, then call me with this."

He sets forth and after some time, meets up with a swarm of bees. He asks the queen bee if perhaps she knows where Rose Maiden lives. The queen bee sends all the other bees in the hive out. They return without any news of where Rose Maiden is. But one bee is still missing. At last she returns and brings with her the eagerly awaited information.

The bee shows the boy the way to Rose Maiden. He finds a place for himself as the goose keeper in the castle where Rose Maiden lives. Every day he sees Rose Maiden. She is as beautiful as milk and blood.

When he hears that Rose Maiden goes to a ball in the city every evening, he rings the bell and calls the woods-woman, his magical foster mother. She gives him a copper horse and a copper cloak, a silver horse and a silver cloak, and a golden horse and a golden cloak so he can attend the ball for three evenings.

While there, he spends all his time talking to Rose Maiden and she enjoys herself greatly. Rose Maiden tells her friends of the beautiful youth and how every night he flies away on his magical horse.

Word of Rose Maiden's interest finds its way to her mother. She tells Rose Maiden a way to discover who the young man is. On the last evening Rose Maiden follows her mother's advice and puts a little tar in his hair.

After the ball, when Rose Maiden searches for her lover, she finally takes a close look at the goose boy and sees that the tar's stuck in *his* hair.

All this while, a dragon has been sleeping in a barrel bound by three rings. But as the young man, Rose Maiden, and her mother fly away on the copper, silver and golden horses, the dragon awakens and the three rings burst from around the barrel.

The dragon flies after, captures them and puts them under a spell. The dragon laughs and says to the boy, "You'll never free Rose Maiden. You could only accomplish that if you had a steed from my mother. And that's impossible."

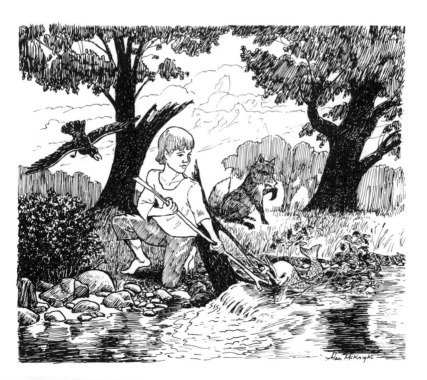

On hearing this the young man shakes off the spell and goes in search of the dragon mother. Along his way, he meets, listens to, and helps a mother raven, a mother fox, and a mother fish. In thanks the raven gives him three feathers, the fox gives him three hairs, and the fish gives him three scales.

When he finds the cottage of the dragon mother, he asks her if she'll take him into her service. "If you agree to one thing," she says after the manner of witches. "Should you ever fail to bring the mare back home again before sunset, you forfeit your life." The witch had already had many in her service. All had failed to return her horse and she killed them all.

On the next day the young man goes out with the mare and the three foals into the meadow. Before he knows it, they've all disappeared. He can't find them by himself, so he rubs together the three feathers and the raven comes, saying, "The mare is among the clouds." So she is. He finds her and brings her home just in time.

On the next day, the mare and her foals disappear again. This time the fox helps him to find her in the depths of the mountains. On the third day the fish helps him find her, for she has fled to the bottom of the sea.

The old dragon mother rubs her eyes in amazement. "Such a one has never been with me before," she thinks.

The year progresses without further event. The old woman and the youth get along well together, and at the end of the year she gives him a foal in thanks.

Given his choice of foals, he takes the weakest, and again the dragon mother is amazed. From whom did he learn that this was the correct one?

Then, of course, the youth and Rose Maiden are united with the aid of the horse and live happily ever after. [Or until their daughter is thirteen.]

I think the following aspects of this tale tell us about dragons and women and blood mysteries.

• The youth is raised by a woods-woman, also known as a wise woman or witch. This means that since the time he was little, he's been acquainted with the ways of nature and how to work with her to accomplish seemingly impossible tasks.

• There are no fathers in this fairy tale. This indicates a matrilineal situation.

• The queen bee symbolizes matriarchal order.

• The mare symbolizes matriarchy and the goddess.

• The Rose Maiden is as beautiful as milk and blood. Together with bee honey, these are the three holy substances of matrilineal cultures.

• The pre-Christian rose is a symbol for blood, love, fertility, and (above all) sensuality. In Christian mysticism the rose characteristically symbolizes the chalice which catches the blood.

• The dragon, guardian of treasures, guards the Rose Maiden, protecting her until the time and circumstances are right. As Rose Maiden's guardian, the dragon also symbolizes the wise use of sexuality, and striking back the unworthy. Many have died by the hand of the dragon mother, because of their inability to pass the tests. The youth does not easily receive the woman of his wishes, nor is he able to simply overpower her. He must undergo tests before he can become one with his beloved. He is able to pass these tests because he was well prepared; he has been brought up in the ways of the Goddess by the woods-woman, who is closely tied to nature, that is, "pagan." In the end the weakest is the strongest.

• He is given a bell. Bells are frequently used to call up ancestral spirits, dakinis, goddesses, and magical beings.

• The boy helps a bird, a fox, and a fish. The triad of the triple goddess/ moon goddess is honored and evoked: the bird of the air/sky/heaven is the maiden; the fox of the earth/mountain is the mother; and the fish of the water/ocean/underworld is the crone. Note also that gold, copper, and silver are symbols for heaven, earth, and water.

• All knowledge and aid comes from mothers and their gifts. Even the animal mothers are helpers in the initiation process. The mother fox, mother raven, and mother fish are wiser than the boy and he is wise enough to use their help. Animals are clever and can help, when one understands their language and honors their abilities.

• The fish and the bottom of the sea are symbols for inner depths and for intuition. The youth must dive deep, gliding far down. He can't force anything, but must simply let himself sink.

• The number three plays a large role. There are *three* horses, *three* rings on the dragon's barrel, *three* mothers (the woods-woman, Rose Maiden's mother, and the dragon mother), *three* magic objects from *three* animals, *three* times the mare disappears with her *three* young ones. Three is the ancient number of the goddess and is often associated with tests in fairy tales. That which is three times fulfilled is final.

• The boy serves the dragon mother a year and a day. This is the minimum time that must pass before an initiate is brought into the magic circle.

• Only when the youth has investigated all three planes will the dragon be satisfied and relinquish Rose Maiden to him. (Note as well that the dragon is satisfied by means of his *mother*'s horse, who gave it to this boy only when she was relatively sure that he had fulfilled all the magic laws.)

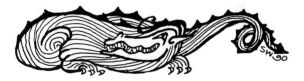

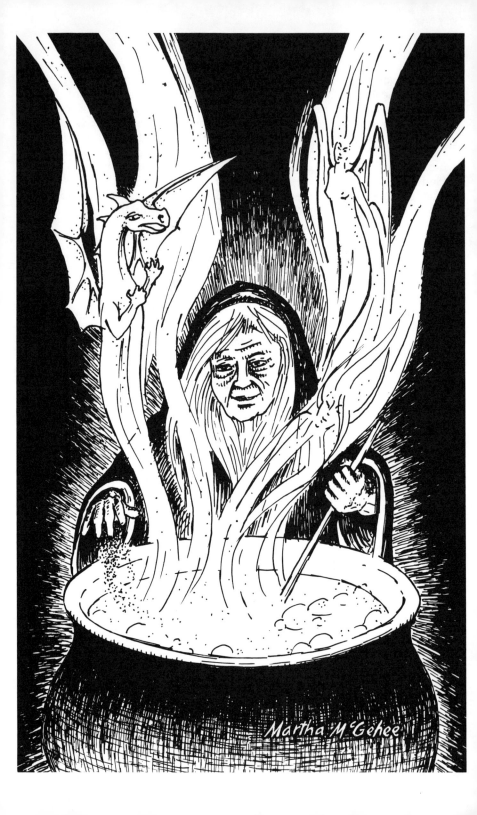

The Cauldron

The cauldron symbolizes the womb, primeval vessel of all life. From it emerges all life and into it everything returns. It stands at the end of time or in the underworld. It is deep and dark. Witches cook their soup in it and goddesses cook up people and animals.

Magic metamorphoses take place in the cauldron. Things are burnt up and reshaped, torn to pieces and made living again.

Sometimes the cauldron is filled with tar and the initiate must submerge herself in the deep black darkness to be renewed. In it, now and then, float arms and legs. There's boiling water and snakes in the cauldron, toads, frogs, crabs, and little children.

The odor of blood issues from the cauldron. It smells of hell, as well as paradise. In fairy tales and Celtic myths apprentices must stir the cauldron, not letting it scorch, and tend the fire underneath it.

The cauldron as womb with its precious blood appears from earliest time in myths and fairy tales.

The Celtic three-fold moon goddess Cerridwen possesses a cauldron where she cooks precious magical herbs. The Celtic magician Taliesin (Merlin) is said to have woven all his magic by virtue of a few drops of elixir received from the goddess's cauldron. (Cerridwen is sometimes depicted with a scythe, as the goddess who decides life and death.)

In the shamanic tales of the Eskimo, a wise woman is required to watch without laughing while Moon Woman dances—or forfeit her life. Moon Woman arrives with a cauldron and spins it around and around. Then she takes out a sickle-shaped woman's knife and dances. When she turns, revealing her hollow back, you must run away, so as not to laugh.

A German fairy tale tells of an old witch who agrees to teach a man magical cooking skills. First, she gives Little Jacob a bowl of soup to eat. The soup tastes both strange and wonderful. Little Jacob is nauseated but can't stop eating. When he's eaten it all, he's changed into a dwarf. Then his lessons begin.

In Shakespeare, the cauldron appears as the instrument of power for three witches, the Wyrd sisters, the equivalents of the three Norns, or the three Fates. In using the cauldron, he evokes its primeval associations as well: woman's power of creation.

In three cauldrons cook the wise blood from which all possible life forms are created.

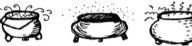

The realm of Dedna (the primeval Eskimo mother) is in the depths of the sea. She can be reached only by passing into an abyss, in the bottom of which turns a slippery and dangerous wheel. Next to the wheel sits a cauldron. Seals cook in the cauldron, being prepared as the spiritual nourishment for humankind.

In the fairy tale *Cook, Little Pot*, the pot is a wonderful source of nourishment, the gift of a goddess. In contrast to other tales, though, the daughter, not the mother, is the one who knows how to use it.

In the fairy tale *The Magic Steed*, a mermaid is brought to the king's castle by a youth versed in magic. She is to marry the king. She orders a great black cauldron to be set up in the courtyard of the castle and has it filled with mare's milk. Then a fire is lit and the milk heated until it begins to foam. The youth and the king are to bathe therein. They shall either be consumed or arise out of the cauldron, born again as higher beings. However, the mermaid is overthrown, the cauldron emptied; the king takes the mermaid and her three enchanted mares into his service. This fairy tale again shows the overthrow of the Goddess and her fertile pot by the patriarchs.

The cauldron gives life and fertility, but the patriarchy fears its power to create change. The tale *King Thrushbeard* describes precisely how the power of the cauldron/woman's belly is to be broken. In the beginning of the story, the princess is pursuing her own desires. She ridicules all suitors, does not want to marry, and criticizes every man who is introduced to her. She's still in a position to take a man of her own choosing.

However, the father figure is already powerful enough to "lay down the law" for his daughter. (As is usual by now, there's no mention of a queen. She's already been disempowered.)

"If you should refuse this next suitor, King Thrushbeard in name, then I swear I'll pledge you to the next beggar," her father says. Still she refuses.

King Thrushbeard (the new hero of a new age) comes disguised in rags as a beggar, intent on breaking the spirit of the princess and taking her into his possession. He'll have her at all costs, but only on his terms.

Once married, he forces her to do house work. She has to weave baskets and do the most menial labor while he is gone all day long. Even though she tries her best, every night he curses her and lays her low.

When he sees that she's almost broken, he has her take, of all things, earthen pots to sell at the market. The symbol of the belly and nourishment is now carried to market by the princess. She manages to find her way there, and the other market women are happy to see her.

Just in the very moment when she's beginning to take some joy in life again, King Thrushbeard rushes in on a horse and breaks her pots to shards. Symbolically speaking, he breaks her will and takes her fertility, her belly, into his possession.

Even this humiliation is not enough. He sends her to his castle to fetch leftovers from a recent wedding celebration. As she fills her little bowl with nourishment (the pot grows ever smaller!) he storms into the hall dressed magnificently, and throws her down so that her bowl falls to the floor, shatters, and all the food spills out. Broken and despairing herself, she's gathering the little shards together when he magnanimously reveals his true identity and offers her a splendid wedding . . . to him . . . the king.

When looking with a dragon's eye, we can see the seizure of power by the patriarchy in this fairy tale. The woman as the cauldron, or pot, is broken. Her womb, her blood, and her life force are taken into men's possession, and from this time forward she is to live tamed and domesticated, reduced to the status of an object, ironically demeaned to status as "vessel" for man.

The cauldron of life then becomes the devil's cauldron, where poor unfortunate souls boil. The primeval mother of life and death becomes a gruesome witch, in whose cauldron little children, toads, and snakes are cooked, a cauldron where enchanted drinks are brewed, brews which turn men to stone or cast a spell over them.

In many ancient temples and ritual sites all over the world, there are chalices, bowl-shaped stones, and vessels meant to hold sacred blood, menstrual blood. In Malta, every temple contains stone chalices and the remnants of red paint. Male priests, lacking their own menstrual blood, substitute "precious life fluid" from sacrificial animals or vanquished enemies. In the matrifocal period, peace was spiritual; now patrifocal religions call for bloody wars.

The Hittites left behind a picture of mother death with a cauldron.

As the female, the empty womb, and menstrual blood all became obscene and were declared taboo, new myths grew. Blood was raised to ethereal heights so it could be borne by men. (How many strong men do you know who faint at the sight of blood? I know many.)

The bleeding belly, center of all life, is renamed "the holy grail" to symbolize spiritual superiority and male enlightenment. The grail is distant and pleasantly unreal. One can search for it forever and yet never have to confront it with the fullness of one's senses, never have to see or smell its bloody contents. Heroic deeds can be undertaken, manly associations founded in the name of the holy grail, keeping women as distant pure *objects*, to be yearned after or fought over. The messy menstruating woman, spreading her odor everywhere, is finally hidden away and separated from Christian spirituality.

The grail was embraced by the educated classes, but the memory of the goddess's cauldron and her fertile blood was too strong among the masses. What could the church offer instead? A goblet containing the blood of the new Hero, Jesus. "He died for you. Worship his blood which he shed for you."

Neither grail nor goblet replaced the cauldron completely. Many people continued to honor the goddess and her fertile cauldron. By the thirteenth century in Europe, the Church was well enough established and rich enough to eliminate these heretics, even using unpopular measures, so the "witches" (women who heal) were brought to "trial." For over 300 years (during the time of the "Gestapo of God," as Barbara Walker calls the Inquisition) witches were tortured and murdered. Any remnants of the old religion were removed from myths and history books, and above all, from the thoughts and feelings of the surviving people.

Though horrible in its consequences (9 million women killed), the Inquisition in Europe deeply imprinted us with certain important symbols and associations:

• The witch's cat. [Everywhere in the ancient world, the lioness was symbol, consort, guardian of the Goddess.]

• The old woman and her constantly boiling and foaming cauldron (the seething womb of life and death).

• The witch's broom. [Her staff of power, representing the sexuality of women, the engulfing vulva, and wild women who made men impotent.] Also see "cleaning fits," p. 33.

• The witch's familiars: toads, snakes and dragons (symbols of birth and menstruation.)

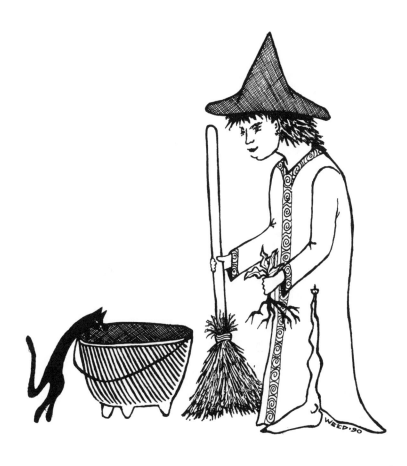

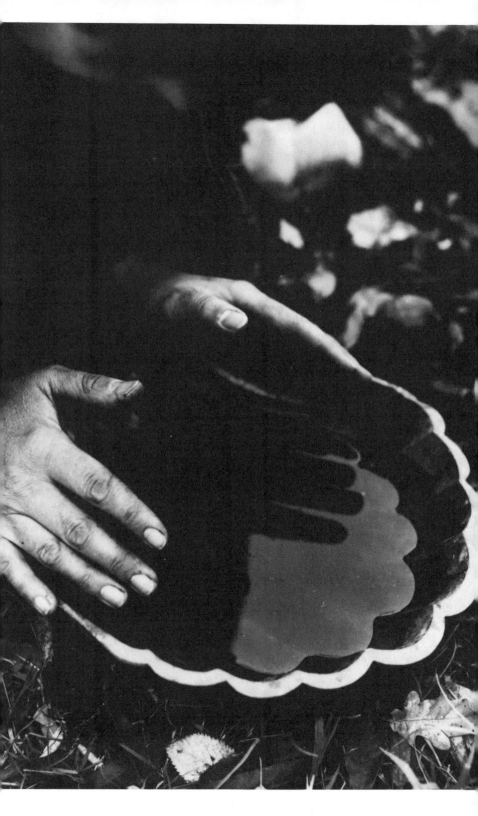

Blood

Menstruation was celebrated before it became taboo. Today hardly any records of these celebrations remain. This revealing account tells of a menstrual festival among the Makonde women in East Africa, which takes place to mark the end of *Unyago*, the time of initiating the newly-bleeding girls of the tribe.

The place of celebration is the open air between the four or five huts of the little hamlet itself. The activity starts about eight in the morning. Old women are busy cleaning the place of celebration with improvised brooms. The young women who will celebrate, are squatting, pressed up close against a wall on the ground in the shadow of a house. They are covering their eyes and temples with their hands and stare unwaveringly through their fingers at the ground.

Suddenly a half dozen women run back and forth across the open area between the houses, making loud trilling noises and other sounds of celebration. This is repeated four or five times. Then the women sing: *Anamanduta nwanangu nwanangwe* (It is going away, it is going away, my dear child), while they cross back and forth across the area three times singing and clapping their hands.

This song is followed immediately by a second song, presented by the same women in the same manner: *Namahihio atjikuta kumaweru.* (The owl hoots in the bush.) Following this song is a remarkable ceremony: women, apparently the teachers of the novices, ornament the girls' heads with bunches of millet. After that, the whole group of women form a line one behind the next. Each woman lays her hands on the shoulders of the one in front, and they all begin to move the middle part of their bodies in a circular motion. Along with that comes the song: *Chihakatu*

29

Cha ruliwili nande kuhuma nchere. (The wicker basket is carried from the house.)
The women bring in gifts from all sides. Millet, *mhogo*, and the like. An egg is cracked and the yolk is smeared on the forehead of the novices. Then an egg is mixed with castor oil and the girls are anointed on breast and back. That is the sign of maturity and with that Unyago is ended. Then the young women who are being celebrated are ornamented and dressed anew. On one spot medicine is buried. This place is marked with a stake. The medicine is a root. In another place a cauldron containing water was buried two months ago.

The continuation of the celebration is announced by the usual trilling, which is such a characteristic display of happiness for East African women, and is therefore heard on all festive occasions. With the trilling there is, implicitly, rhythmic clapping of hands. Along with the continuing trilling and hand clapping another song is sung. *Kanole wahum kwetu likundasi kugeidya ingombo.* (Have a look at the girl. She's borrowed the string of pearls and doesn't yet know what to do with it.) This song is followed quickly by another: *Ignole yangala mene mtuleke weletu tuwakuhiyo loka.* (You, you there, who are together in the *Unyago*, be happy, celebrate. We, we here, who have come to you, we have no wish to play along, just to watch.)

Then follows a long pause, at the end of which the women line up again to the right, and wedged between them stand the young women of the celebration. They are now totally wrapped up. With garishly colored new cotton cloth over their head and upper body they now look like moving bundles of cloth. In slow rhythm and to the beat of the drums they sing their song while they edge forward into the middle of the area of celebration. While doing so, they all move their midriffs again in lively circles.

Then slowly the circle of women drifts apart. The oldest of the women stands in the middle and in front of her step, one by one, the novices. Now it is their duty to show, in front of the severe crone, what they have learned in the isolation of their long *Unyago* lessons: it is a parallel to the trilling already described, only instead of the tongue, now the rear end moves in quick trembling motion back and forth.

Again everyone breaks formation. Then, at a rapid pace, although in short tip-toe steps, a bundle of clothes breezes into the middle. It is a woman. Standing out large and white is the *Pelele*, the lip ornament on the brown face. She opens the dance for the entire village. (Dr. B. Shidlof, Berlin 1925)

Unyago, the time of learning and growing for girls, still exists in some tribes. Among the Agni of Ghana and the Ivory Coast, at the time of their first menstruation, girls are initiated into the art of healing with herbs, spending eight months with the medicine woman. Then, rubbed with ashes, they dance their initiation dance with their teachers. There are surprising parallels between these puberty dances of the young women in Africa and Women's Fasching dances in Germany and Austria.

H. P. Duerr describes in *Traumzeit (Dreamtime)*, women tearing their bonnets from their heads at Fasching celebrations specifically for women and dancing around half naked and with their hair loose. Austrian Fasching celebrations include dances with wild, whiplike motions and rapid running in place by women naked from the waist down. The women kindle each other with bundles of barley and likely help young stragglers along with their fingers. In Bulgaria such festivals (often known as midwifery festivals) end with the whole group of women sleeping together. In Forno di Canale, above Belluno, the custom at Women's Fastnacht (Shrove Tuesday) is to have a chime or bell ringing. This reminds us of the use of the bell as a magical tool to call up ancient ones and wise women.

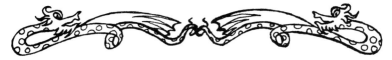

The Catholic church gives us interesting references to the mighty blood of women. Mary's "immaculate" conception doesn't deny the need of the semen and man, but invents the pure Maria, unstained by unspeakable blood.

In eastern Europe, the custom still remains of announcing a young woman's first menses by hanging the stained bedsheet out the window.

And what of the tongues of fire at Pfingsten (Pentacost)? Drops or tongues of fire are said to have fallen from heaven then and to have put the people into a trance. In reality there are pagan customs in which menstrual blood (mixed with water) is sprinkled to hypnotize, heal, or cast spells.

> Should a witch be known to have taken part in an imaginary or real celebration, either by being denounced, or because her name was forced out of a fellow sufferer under torture, or because she herself revealed having been there, then she paid with death by fire. But the fire itself was said to have already flamed up in her. Over it boiled and bubbled her cauldron. She watched over it and guarded it. (Duerr, *Traumzeit*.)

Producing heat in the body is one method of preparing for ecstasy. The crafts of healing and magic are also thought of as a heat.

> Woman appears as the guardian of fire. Hers is the fire of below, earth fire, differing from the fire that falls from heaven, lightning, the masculine fire, which can be bored out of wood. Also the libido—flaming up as sexuality, the inner fire, leading to orgasm and in the orgasm of ecstasy finding its higher expression—is in this sense a fire reposing in woman and simply set in motion by the male. The sign of female ardor, the trail of blood which the male no longer sniffs after, nose to the ground, is menstruation. Red is the color of fire and blood. Young witches have red hair, and amid a raging fire, they burn on the funeral pyre. (Annemarie Dross, *Die erste Walpurgisnacht* [*The First Walpurgis Night*], Frankfurt, 1978.)

I know of depictions of goddesses uncovering their vulva and sending forth the streaming odor of their blood, putting the fear of death into men and sending them into flight. Once again, this gesture finds refuge in lewd dances done by women.

In the (truly idiotic) book by George Devereux, *Baubo. Die mythische Vulva* (*The Mythical Vulva*), Frankfurt, 1981—which would be better named "Mystification of the Penis," there is one single, and therefore very interesting reference to the meaning of menstruation, which otherwise never appears, although the theme of the book is vulva.

Curious that Devereux, a psychoanalyst, doesn't recognize the connection to menstrual envy. "In Central Australia the subincised adult handles his (split) urethra as though it were a vagina. In certain rites he makes it bleed and so imitates the menstruation of women."

It's remarkable that Devereux, as well as other authors who bandy female sexuality and its taboos about so freely, largely ignore menstruation or handle it in as clinical and distant a manner as possible. While every possible form of coitus between human and animal, mortal and god, or god and goddess is covered without restraint, the embarrassing blood is left out. Anxiety raised by the bleeding woman is deeply rooted and stimulated by even the slightest of allusions.

Men's menstrual angst has led them to try to isolate women and shut them out of life, society, and "his-tory." Menstrual huts, once places of power where women celebrated and held rituals together, became prisons. In South America, menstruating indigenous women now go into a tiny hut alone, squat over certain leaves, and there squeeze out their blood. These leaves are burned and buried in a place removed from the village, instead of honored as fertile, life-giving, and holy.

Mana radiates from a woman when she is bleeding: a dangerous power, according to some Indonesians.

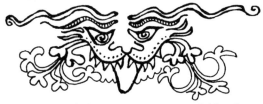

The special powers of dragontime menstrual blood, once used so skillfully by associations of women, are still feared today by the patriarchs. Their ways and rules encourage women to misdirect this power into self-loathing, into pain and depression and moodiness, into buying crazes and the compulsion to shoplift, into fits of despair. But women can still find and use this power. And those who do are no longer tame nor helpless in the face of destructive male rage.

Cleaning fits during or before menstruation have been much abused and ridiculed. Their mythical meaning? In Africa, sweeping and cleaning to scare off "demons" is still a custom. During menstruation, many women are especially sensitive, accessible, vulnerable, all the more so if out of touch with their own blood power. And so it is that inner feelings of chaos, pain, aggression, and anxiety become demons. By sweeping away the outer demons and purifying the outer world we hope to find inner peace and respite from the inner dragons.

As we read in the account from Africa, the custom at the beginning of the menstrual celebration is to have old women (those, so to speak, who are experienced in dealing with demons) sweep the ceremonial site.

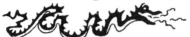

The Stone Age rock paintings in France, Spain, the Dolomites, the Tassili Mountains of Algeria, Air Mountains of Nigeria, and elsewhere allude to the power of bleeding women: they are all done in red. Depictions of red hands (bloody hands) are common. Even more frequent are vaginas of all sorts painted in red.

The female gender and figurines of women are central to the entire early history of the world. In her books, *The Goddesses and Gods of Old Europe*, and *The Language of the Goddess*, Marija Gimbutas describes the many different kinds of vessels, vulva-like bowls, cauldrons, goddess figurines, and female idols that tell us of women's fertility, blood, birth, and power.

The color red played a vital role in early societies. Up to this day it retains its meaning as the color of life. Contracts are sealed in blood.

Female bleeding was the only sure and dependable thing in the life of the clan, coming and going as regularly as the moon.

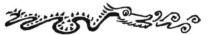

In tantric teachings, a menstruating woman is considered a most precious partner. With her one can experience the essence of womanliness itself, and know the power of woman.

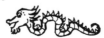

Blood is our trail. If we follow this red thread into the labyrinth, then we will surely encounter our power.

The Tuareg women in the Tassili Mountains of Algeria, where I spent some time, showed me how they handle the menstrual flow without using pads or tampons. (They live so removed from supplies that our usual consumption of sanitary products is simply not possible, if only because of the difficulties of transportation and storage.)

At the beginning of menstruation they separate themselves from the rest of the family and squat over a hole which they've dug in the earth. They allow the first flow of blood to run out, then tense their muscles to hold it in. During the menstruation, there are times when they bleed and times when they do not. They sense it and regulate it. If now and then some blood drips, they simply spread their legs wide. They wear no underpants. The light odor of stale blood common among Europeans never occurs among them. The air can reach the vagina at all times. Every now and then, they jump and move around playfully to air out their vaginas.

They're very open about their sexuality. Not only do they kiddingly stroke and touch themselves (and me) with a mixture of sensuality and lust, they also dance (always on a Thursday evening) searching out new partners or coming on to old ones, baring their sexual parts, and laughing long and loud.

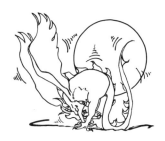

Bloody Stories

Many traces of what was once surely the original power of blood have been left to us in old stories and fairy tales. In them, the most important magical substance of all is blood. Even a single drop of blood can have great power: the ability to speak, to see, and to remember.

In stories and fairy tales, it is blood that reveals the murderer, blood that curses, blood that awakens, blood that enchants. In one story, an underwordling is called to earth by means of blood. (He marries, but his sojourn on earth is short: he treats his wife badly and she returns to the home of her mother and sister. Unavoidably, this reminds me of the dull but numerous jokes where a woman packs her bags and goes back to mother. Seen in a different light, these jokes address women's sovereignty in matrifocal situations and how the patriarchy tries to make this look ridiculous.)

Blood can make you see again. It can heal warts and wounds, drive out spirits, or bind them to you. Pacts with the devil are sealed in blood. And what is written in blood is good for all eternity. Blood is the seat of the soul, the continuation of the family. Indeed, "families" can even be created by the physical act of mixing blood from a cut or wound: so it was that the men of blood brotherhoods were tied to one another, mimicking the primeval sisterhoods of menstruation.

The power of all blood derives from the power of menstrual blood. When we understand how aware people were of menstrual blood since prehistoric times, and how recently this memory has sunk out of awareness, then we can read fairy tales with new understanding.

Cinderella

A rich man, widowed and with a younger daughter, remarries and the woman brings her two daughters with her into the marriage. The daughters are beautiful of face but ugly of heart and mean-spirited with the man's daughter, soon known only as Cinderella.

As it so happens, at the time when all are old enough to marry, the prince of the land is also seeking a wife. The king holds three gala balls. Cinderella, denied permission to attend the balls by her stepmother, pulls from three magic hazel nuts three wonderful dresses with matching shoes and a coach, and goes to the balls in secret. The three dresses are the color of the sea (the unconscious), the color of the heavens (the flight of the soul), and the color of fire (the womb, menstrual blood, fertility and passion).

The prince will dance with no one but Cinderella. On the first and second night, she leaves at the end of the ball without event. But on the last evening, wearing the dress the color of fire, Cinderella loses her shoe as she runs away. [Because the prince has coated the stairs with pitch!]

According to *The Pocket Dictionary of German Superstitions*, the shoe (like the cauldron) symbolizes the womb or vagina. So we may surmise that what she actually "lost" was her virginity (giving a much more suggestive cast to the prince's subsequent search of the shoe that "fits").

When the prince's quest for his beloved takes him at last to Cinderella's house, the stepsisters try to fool him, by cutting their feet to fit into the shoe. But blood begins to ooze out of the shoe. (They are menstruating.) Only Cinderella's foot fits without a drop of blood. (She is pregnant.)

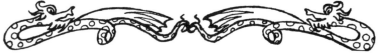

The power of blood in European fairy tales coincides with the beneficence and power associated with the color red in India. Kali-Maya (the Crone and Dancer) and the creative nourishing energy of her menstrual blood are evoked by dying cloth red, by painting hands and feet with red patterns, and by daubing the forehead with red powder.

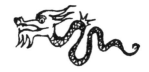

Acacia gum, which is gathered from the African desert acacia, is also known as "clots of menstrual blood." It has important functions in healing and magic. Acacia itself stands for woman.

In voodoo cults, fetish amulets can be powerful only when properly treated with blood, preferably menstrual blood. Many times, the women who make blood amulets are called witches.

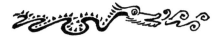

Egyptian Pharaohs had to drink the "blood of Isis," a fluid named *sa*, in order to become holy and powerful.

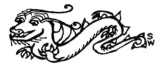

The vampire sucks the blood out of a victim (often a woman) and so receives the strength to live, the life force taken directly, not as flesh or milk, but as original nourishment: blood. [A story about a vampire who specifically sought menstrual blood appeared recently in an American woman's magazine.]

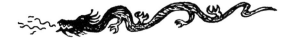

In Celtic Britain, the color red was both the symbol of earthly power and of divine selection by the goddess.

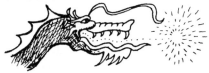

One need not look too deeply into the myth of the goddess Cybele to see her frequent connections to caves and the color red, that is, the womb and menstrual blood.

Nor is the symbolism of this very old Greek legend too difficult to discern: the Thessalian witch (woman of power and wisdom) gathers moon drops (menstrual blood) at the dark of the moon (when women not exposed to artificial light would be menstruating). Her most powerful medicine/poison is made with the moon drops shed by the woman-no-longer maiden, who bleeds for the first time. About these moon drops there is a strong taboo.

A Chinese myth describes the goddess Chang-O who guards the menstrual blood. When she lived on earth, men attacked her. They envied her bleeding, for it meant that she possessed the power of life, death, and rebirth, and these were mysteries to them. She became so angry at the men's jealous attacks that she herself withdrew to the moon and forbade men to take part in her festivals from then on. So it came to be that in China, the women celebrate full moon festivals only among themselves, with songs and praise to honor women and Chang-O and menstrual blood, the blood of life and death.

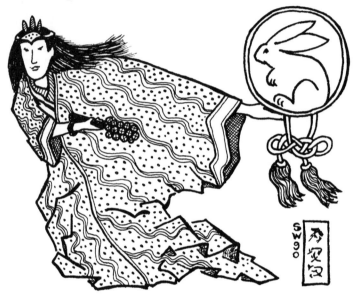

Australian aborigines paint their cult stones with red earth and call them "menstrual blood of women."

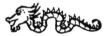

The water of life and death reconnects us to the European fairy tales, where the hero/ine, in search most often of the beloved, is led by three witches, or a dragon grandmother, or perhaps an old aunt (one of the ancient ancestors), to a spring which wells with the water of life and death. Drinking, sucking, licking up the welling spring water, bathing in, anointing with, sprinkling on the living water, the hero/ine is nourished, renewed, and made wiser.

When we rediscover the importance of our menstrual blood, as well as our entire menstrual cycle (with its three phases—maiden, mother, crone—into which this bleeding divides our womanly life), we hear familiar tales in new ways, as, for instance, these favorites.

Rose Red, Briar Rose, or Sleeping Beauty

A queen and her king/consort are eager for children but unable to conceive. Her ardent desire stirs the fairies [in some versions, the "wise women"] to aid her. One day she bathes in a pond where a frog lives (frogs are one of the most ancient symbols of fertility, birthing women, and the vagina) and is told she'll bear a child. Her pregnancy comes through ancient powers, mythical powers, woman-centered powers.

Despite this, after she gives birth, the baptismal party proceeds in the spirit of the patriarchy. Instead of thirteen silver plates (which represent the unique lunar year) the table is set with twelve golden plates (which represent the divisible, repeatable solar year) and only twelve fairies [or wise women] are invited . . . the "good" ones.

The thirteenth fairy, betrayed and grieving, comes to the baptismal party and appears to curse the infant girl with death (the symbolic death of woman in patriarchal society). Thirteen is the number of death, metamorphosis, and rebirth, tying it into the menstrual cycle's ever-changing flow of growth, dissolution, and regeneration.

Rose Red is to prick her finger on a spindle [bleed] and die before she turns fifteen. [Fifteen years is the age of initiation into adulthood, the average age of menstrual onset for women not exposed to artificial light.] The last fairy to be invited has one wish left and she changes the death into a one hundred year sleep.

Amusingly enough, and evidence of how magic can't be avoided, the adults guard Rose Red closely throughout her childhood, but relax their efforts on her fifteenth birthday. On that day, Rose Red makes her way to the tower (often a place of initiation for women, as in the tale of Rapunzel). [In blood mysteries, towers do not represent sexual initiation or a phallus, but the ability of the menstruating woman to have a wide overview of the possibilities.]

In the tower time stands still, representing the time between childhood and womanhood when a woman lives between the worlds until she knows who she is. There sits an ancient woman spinning. (Spinning is one of the oldest symbols for female wisdom. The way a spider spins her thread, weaves her web, and watches it disintegrate, is like a woman creating a womb full of blood-rich nourishment and watching it flow out from between her legs. With the red thread of menstrual wisdom, a woman finds her way in the labyrinth of her inner world, her womanly body.)

Rose Red, who has never seen a spindle [in the patriarchy, the wise ways of women are outlawed, banned, reviled, thought dangerous], grabs it, sticks herself, and—as the blood wells up—sinks into a deep sleep, taking everyone in the castle with her. (She begins her menstruation and is initiated into the secrets of bleeding by the crone. The crone, as embodiment of the matriarchy—where women are not overpowered and taken, but approached with honor—knows that much time must pass before men will once again feel their way toward women and their secrets to heal themselves and their hearts.)

Around the tower grow roses (symbolizing fertility, sexuality, and woman spirit) thick with thorns. Those who approach and thrash about with swords (symbolizing here aggressive masculine sexuality) are entangled and cannot penetrate.

Only the one who approaches with sensitivity passes unharmed, the thorns miraculously change to multicolored flowers. His kiss—of wonder, not possessive passion—awakens the slumbering maiden. [The thirteenth fairy, the wise woman, and the old spinster wink and grin at each other, and quietly merge with Rose Red.]

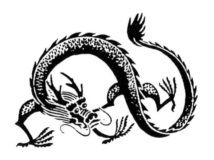

Everyday Blood

See nothing, hear nothing, say nothing, and above all, smell nothing. That's the attitude modern society takes towards menstruation.

Advertisements for pads and tampons are as "tastefully" done as those for toilet paper and other human dirt. In the damp Toilet Paper Culture, where bathrooms and kitchens are equally gleaming, and there's no mention of excrement, tampons and pads are bloomingly white, sterile, clean, and free of mucous, at least metaphorically speaking. (Though the tampon which protects the world from stinking bleeding women can be lethal to women—if it harbors bacteria.)

Advertisements for "sanitary protection" strive to make us feel insecure when we bleed or sweat. In fact, we're so conditioned that we do indeed want most especially not to be noticed doing *such things.*

"Because you wear them on the inside, no one can smell or see a thing." No one else? Or you? Who doesn't want to see or smell a thing?

"The dryer you feel, the better you feel," says an ad for sanitary pads in England. And how does a fish feel on dry land?

What wonderful ideas advertisements give us about ourselves. Madison Avenue assures us that there's no reason for women to be handicapped by menstruation. No reason for women to look any less attractive, stay home, or feel any less confident.

Indeed not, for women are supposed to be the perfectly functioning work force of modern industrial companies. And the tendency is to take the computer as a model for this perfect workforce. Computers are so reliable, so predictable. They don't have migraines, don't talk too much (not at all unless asked), don't sweat, don't need any bathroom or meal breaks, don't menstruate, and don't get PMS: Pre-Menstrual Syndrome. Compared to computers, women are a real pain. They've hardly recovered from menstruating, when they're ovulating—so moody and sexually aggressive. Then comes PMS and the raging need to clean, clean, clean, and to sleep alone, alone, alone. Talk about unpredictable!

Menstruation is a special time, a time when all sorts of energies stream through us. In German computer centers and pharmaceutical labs, menstruating women wear a red dot on their lab coats and are not allowed into certain areas.

What, I ask, are women remembering when they get into those heavy depressions, those outbursts of tears, the sudden acts of aggression, the lingering melancholies? What's going on in our deepest souls when we turn away from our lovers, when we become nauseated, and have to crawl into bed *alone* with cocoa?

Could it be we remember another time? The dog in the apartment still tramples down imaginary grass, turning, turning, before laying to rest. Could it be that menstruation touches on a primal experience, which shines through dimly when the body is in a certain chemical state? And what is it about the pineal gland and this mysterious hormone melatonin that the body produces mainly at night? Does it bring on depression on dark days, or produce dreams in the dark of night?

What's known about melatonin now is that it's produced in greater quantities when the day is dull. From that, the conclusion's been drawn that it's the cause for people's bad moods and depressions on such days.

Of course, in this age of the sun calendar and worshiping of light, it's no wonder we have trouble with the moon and with darkness. Couldn't it be that this hormone has some other use? That melatonin is vital to us for dreaming, for envisioning, spinning tales, remembering?

Women who have migraines (and the odd male sufferer) seek out darkness and avoid bright light. Women with strong psychic and spiritual abilities often seek out darkness.

Caves are the ritual sites for menstruating women. Caves block out the light of day. These are places of menstrual energy, menstrual power, menstrual remembering. [In the dark, the blood mysteries come back to you. Sit quietly, bleeding, and open yourself to the memories.] Menstrual energy is moon energy, is the energy of the night and darkness. There's no room for it in big bright offices, or neon-lit night clubs and metropolitan streets, in factories, department stores, and supermarkets overflowing with light and stimulation. This deep, dark energy of woman fits worst of all into the brightly lit office of the obstetrician, on whose chair a woman may so easily lose her sense of self worth.

Under these circumstances isn't it kindness to take away this burden on woman so she won't always be remembering these vague powers, so she doesn't have to suffer so? Let's take everything out of peoples' minds that makes them unable to function. Let's free them from these useless sensations, running through them like pain in an amputated leg.

Menstruation is superflous now. Away with it, for then "this day will be like all days for you." Or at least gulp down your daily Pill and enjoy a pretty little menstruation: punctual, painfree, and regular. "Then you won't ever need to pass up fun," says a tampon advertisement. The only intelligent question I've found in all the tampon and pad commercials is: "Have you every wondered how men would hold up if they had your periods?"

An English firm admits it can't "make a laughing matter out of your period," but "we can make it less of a bloody nuisance." When I read the word bloody in this context, I have to think of "bloody Mary" and the immaculate conception. At a place of pilgrimage dedicated to Maria, I celebrate bloody Mary and drink a sip of holy water to her and to my bloody health.

Many women in the past hundred years have lost their uterus (and ovaries) to male-dominated medical thinking. After all, "they aren't actually necessary to a woman's well-being" (although the operation does indeed seem to be necessary to the gynecologist's well-being), and "you'll finally be free of your bloody monthly mess."

But if you're not quite ready to go that far, then sometimes the thought will wander through your mind that menstruation/dragontime is a special time, when all sorts of things are going on for you.

You can ignore these things, look the other way, grit your teeth and go on "in spite of them." You can celebrate them, too.

Begin by noticing your dragontime. Pick up the trail of this energy by keeping a menstrual diary. Get an overview of how you feel in different situations when you bleed. What goes well? What goes poorly? How's menstruation in the summer? Winter? On bright days? On dull ones? Is bad weather just right to help you get through? What's too much for you? What do you need more of?

Note how your menstruation swings softly back and forth between full moon and new moon, waning moon and waxing moon, or how it occurs at the same moon phase or in the same astrological sign. Discover how year after year, your bleeding occurs in a special dance with the moon.

Do even more. When you menstruate (preferably on the first night), go out and look for the moon. Get a star chart and have someone show you how to find the different constellations. Observe also if the moon is sliding through the Pleiades, or touching, covering, or passing a planet. Gather all these heavenly sights and sensations as you bleed and get in touch with how you feel.

To get in touch with your dragontime power, focus a ritual celebration around it. (Menstrual blood carries a strong emotional charge and changes every ritual. It's good if women know each other well and trust each other before doing such work for a lot of energy will be freed up, and may emerge passionately.)

Gather with the other women who are menstruating at the same time in the woods (in summer) or in a well-heated room (in the winter). Drink red juice or wine. Paint yourself with blood or red paint. Stamp or clap or beat a basic rhythm (see p. 79). Let each woman in turn come into the circle and dance the feeling that's released by her menstruation: jumping, swaying, drooping, standing still, cowering, hopping, stomping. While each dances out what she feels, the others keep the beat constant.

When all have danced, join hands, stand, and lean softly to and fro. Let each woman take up energy from the swaying movement of the one next to her and pass it on. To open this circle, each woman covers her solar plexus with both hands.

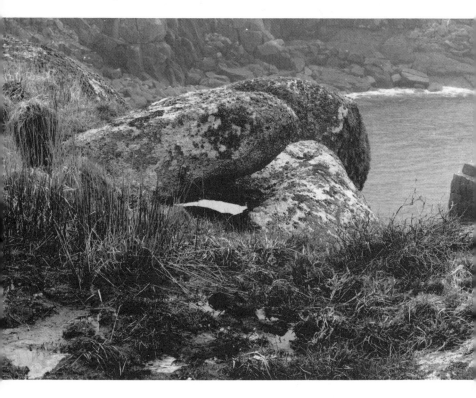

Oh, dragonblood, what are your powers?
What can this dragonblood do?

Turn clean white pads *red*.
Turn women into dragons.
That's what I do.

DRAGONTIME
Menstrual Magic

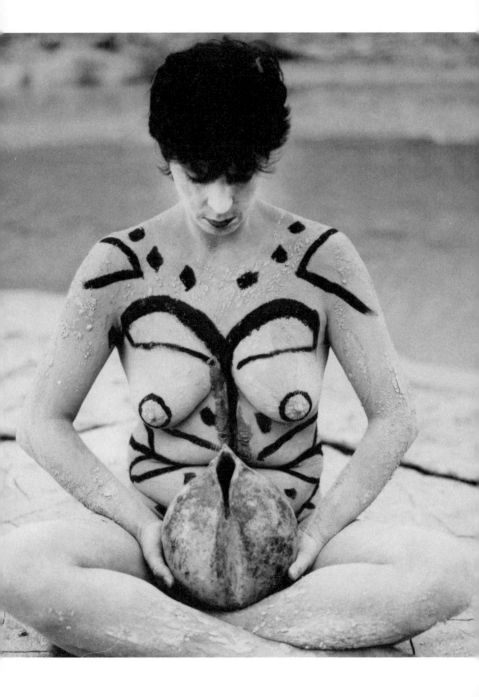

Menstrual Magic:
Using Our Dragontime Abilities

Once we realize that menstruation is a special time, our dragontime, then it's easy to see that it's also a time of special powers. Even if never recognized or used, they reside in all women as potential: magical, fierce, wonderful.

As is the case with all magical and mythical processes, there are particular stones, plants, animals, and other allies which harmonize with the vibration of menstruation and open our channels. As metaphors and as realities, these allies show us ways of wisdom, power, and magic.

To receive the gifts of these messengers, to become adept at menstrual magic, we need to learn other languages. A stone can't speak like a person. An animal won't set itself in front of you and say, "Here are three hairs. When you rub them together, you'll call me and I'll help you."

How can we learn the magical language of dragontime? There are many ways. Spending time in my menstrual hut is my favorite way. There I rearrange my altar, write in my moon book, and reconnect with my allies. Some of my other favorites are: relaxing, reading oracles, talking to myself, dreaming, going on trance journeys, dancing and creating rituals.

Deep relaxation eases physical pain, is mentally calming, and emotionally soothing. As a prelude to trance journeys, or as a separate practice, deep relaxation awakens the "inner senses" which "speak dragon."

When I began to work with menstruation, I went into a deeply relaxed state to release my belly cramps and find out where they were coming from. Initially when I relaxed fully, I experienced a wonderful feeling of lightness.

Then, suddenly, I felt like someone was bandaging me and laying me in a stone coffin. I couldn't move. I almost panicked. I wasn't able to deal with the feeling so I tried to sit up, but I couldn't move my legs. It was like I was paralyzed. Then it dawned on me: I did the same thing to my womb, zipping it into tight jeans, sucking it in all the time because I didn't want to have a belly at all. Bellies are so fat and burdensome.

I had done my relaxation by candle light, and had filled a bamboo cup with water before I went into the trance. As I made the connection to my constricted belly, the bamboo cup broke into two pieces and I could move my legs again! I felt incredibly free. The two halves of the bamboo cup on my altar now remind me of my flash of insight.

Another ancient method for learning magical languages is talking to yourself. More specifically, concentrate on a plant, an object, an animal, or take a hike in the mountains, float in a boat on the water, or stare into a fire and begin to talk "emptily." Let your mouth become a channel for energy, for messages.

Many women talk to themselves and are embarrassed about it. But it's an important way to pick up on vibrations and make them audible, palpable, real. Conversing with yourself makes audible to you the old speech. I listen for the old language, the body language, the uncensored tongue, when I sing and talk to myself.

Another way to talk to yourself is to play this association game, which can be done alone or with a group of women.

Association Game

Take a big piece of paper, and starting at the top middle, write a word you want to begin with, for instance: "BLOOD." Under it, draw a line to the left and one to the right and associate two words, for instance, "mess" and "pain." With both of these words, write two more that you associate with each of them. A mountain emerges, built from the top down. The game is half over when there's no more room on the right and left of the paper, and a mountain or triangle of words and phrases has been created.

Then form sentences, however you like, out of all the words in your triangle. The only words you may use that aren't in the triangle are linking words, for instance, and/or/on. These sentences will lead you to your deepest memories. At the beginning, it seems totally ridiculous, then it becomes an amazing experience, leading you to hidden parts of yourself.

To do it with others, sit in a circle, shut your eyes, and have everyone speak, one by one. Each woman speaks a word that she associates with menstruation. Continue going around until no more words come. Keep silent afterwards for a few minutes letting everything circle around. Then make sentences.

To avoid women talking too long or too much, pass around a talking stick. You may speak only when you have the stick.

[The menstruating woman, from the vantage point of her tower, can "see the future"—as well, of course, as the past and the present. Ancient oracles, such as the one at Delphi, were "staffed" by bleeding women. You can prophesy for yourself in many ways and so learn more of the language of dragontime.]

When you're bleeding, set an object you've chosen across from you and feel your way into it. Open yourself to the validity of all your impulses and thoughts, all the associations which go through your head. Ask it a question and read the signals that arise in you.

Go outside with your question. You will be led to your oracle. Many answers can be found in nature.

Visions and dreams, including daydreams, are keys to the language of dragontime. To find these keys, keep a dream diary. Note your feelings, colors or symbols you see, animals and plants that come to you in dreams whenever you can. [Daydreams, also known as visions, are vivid, oracular, and exceptionally accessible during the first several days of a woman's menstrual flow. Bleeding-time dreams, visions, inspirations, and feelings are often visual, sensual, detailed, and emotionally charged.]

Like dreams and visions, guided visualizations and trance journeys help us hear with the inner ear and be quiet enough to perceive the shy inner wisdom. [Trance journeys help me remember my dragontime abilities when I'm not bleeding, and expand them when I am.]

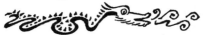

Another magical, mythical, embodied way of learning the language of Dragontime is to dance. Menstrual dragon dances may have been the very first dances as women swayed serpentlike together to ease the pelvis, hips, thighs, belly engorged with blood.

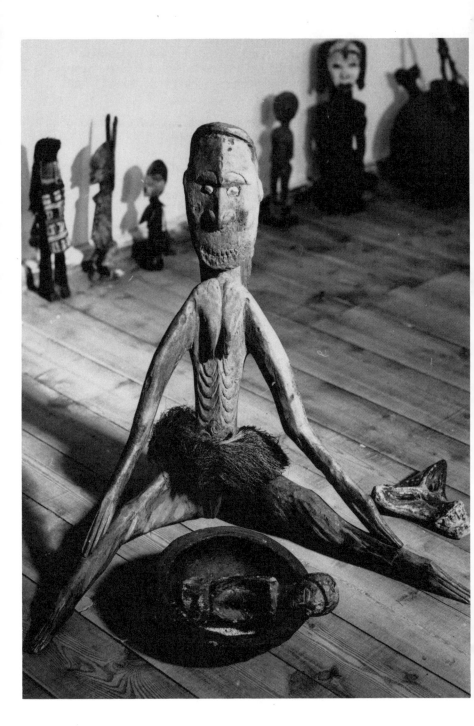

Menstrual Huts and Dragon Lairs

A New Guinea aborigine killed his wife after she slept on his blanket during menstruation. He thought there was no other way to avoid her frightening and harmful influence.

Males of many cultures exhibit a psychotic fear of "mana," the incalculable power of women during their bleeding. In the face of this it's no wonder that a place which is so important for women, their own space, the menstrual hut, becomes a place of exile.

My initial knowledge of menstrual huts came from Native American and African cultures where the huts isolate women during their bleeding time.

Yet, when I tried it, I found that having a menstrual space is truly a wonderful thing, a place into which I could withdraw and feel protected.

My first menstrual space was the spare room of a city apartment where I lived. It was carpeted; the floor was warm and soft. All my favorite stones were there, as well as figurines of different goddesses, and a few little clay figures of women, given to me by my friends. Besides that, a few shells, candles and soft pillows.

When I'd bleed, I'd go to this room, taking a blanket, a hot water bottle, a mug of cocoa, perhaps a trashy novel. Here I could dream, meditate, ruminate undisturbed, and find peace. After awhile, I began to seek out this sacred little room at times other than menstruation.

Since moving to the land, I've built myself a moon hut, a dragon lair of seven tall wooden poles with blankets and cloth thrown over to make a cave/tent. The floor is covered with cronewort (mugwort/*Artemisia vulgaris*). Inside I can make a little fire and, with a nice mat to lay on,

I can sleep there even on damp days. I love having a place that reminds me of the power of my menstruation.

I do rituals there. Sometimes I go into a trance. I write down my bleeding time visions and images; often I can develop these into real plans and weave them into my daily life.

During menstruation, I'm especially drawn to a few particular holy springs. I won't name these places because I don't believe in giving "travel tips"; you can find similar places on your own. Look for springs near little chapels or by caves. They often have folk names like "Mary's" or "Women's," "Hell's" or "Witches." The Goddess is alive at these holy places, women's ancient places of power.

I've also experimented with bowl-shaped stones, and drawn the conclusion that at least some of them were used in the context of menstruation. With fear of making good anthropologists howl, still I must confess that it's very exciting to engage in little rituals in places already enlivened by folklore [that is, ancient healing/ritual sites].

How wonderful if all women could have menstrual huts, if we could have a room in each community for the use of menstruating women. It would be a haven, a meeting point, a safe space to be during one's period. I envision such a space as comfortable and cozy, with lots of pillows and blankets, things for making herb teas and cocoa (but not coffee, as it stimulates and intensifies bleeding). Soup simmers in a big pot.

Women who come there write in menstrual diaries. Besides the personal diaries, there's a collective book where every woman can add her bleeding time feelings, dreams, and problems. I also envision regular meetings (at the full moon?) where women talk about their bleeding, share their difficulties and good times, celebrate together and create rituals to change the dynamic of their menstruation.

These menstrual huts/dragon lairs are well heated, when necessary, for warmth is very important. An open fire is especially nice: outdoors, even a small one, indoors, in a cookstove or fireplace.

Decorations change and flow like the women's menses. The things around the room are strongly connected to menstruation: cloths and goblets the color of the sea and of blood; pictures of goddesses connected to blood, fertility, and healing; wonderful vulva-like stones and pieces of wood; shells, and bowls of water; red velvet.

And, what for me is the most important thing in a menstrual hut, or any ritual space: the altar.

Menstrual Altars

A lot of women have altars without even knowing it. They collect a couple of stones, some feathers and seashells, a child's shoe, an old photo, a ticket from an important trip, and so on, on their desk. And when they look at them, they feel the warmth of pleasant memories. The power of memories or the association between symbolic objects and your own feelings is the basis for altars, as well as amulets and ritual objects.

When you begin your menstrual altar, think over which objects you want to use and what you want to express. Try to clearly identify the many powers and feelings you want to include.

I have an old chest inherited from an aunt in which I save stones, shells, feathers, herbs and magical objects. Everything that goes into my chest becomes charged. It's made of wood, inlaid with mother-of-pearl birds. It is the base of my menstrual altar; I lay my menstrual power objects on top of the chest.

First, there's a piece of leopard skin I got from an African hunter, who stole it from a white, big-game hunter, feeling that it should belong to me. On top of that, I have a big South Seas shell that roars like the ocean when you hold it up to your ear. And a stone from the Sahara that looks like vulva and has a tiny white pebble caught between its lips. Then there's a little root creature which looks like a dragon. In front of it, I've laid various red beads of carnelian, coral, agate, and garnet. There's a little container made of camel skin, filled with cowrie shells, cronewort (mugwort) and lady's mantle. Two gorgeous, dried, red orchid blossoms sit there, along with a wood carving from Sumatra showing two dragons, red and green, wound around each other, and on top of them, a woman, a dragon rider. Sometimes I add a rag with some blood. Recently my altar included a piece of dried Fly Amanita from a "witches' ring" near Ostern Lake in Bavaria. (A witches' ring is a circle of Fly Amanita, a distinctive, poisonous, red-capped, white-dotted mushroom.)

Menstrual altars look different month to month, woman to woman. Don't limit yourself. Only by trying things out can you decide what belongs there, what gives you energy, what holds good memories. I've used pieces of cloth and wood, symbolic items, wool threads, shells, stones, dolls, pearls, feathers, fish and animal bones, pictures, beads, herbs. What things will your menstrual altar hold?

> • Traditional African amulets for strenghtening woman's power, such as cowrie shell necklaces or leather necklaces with spiral shaped limestone, are wonderful altar pieces. They were once used as currency in West Africa.
> • Red glass beads, red wood beads, red seeds, and dried red fruit can be strung into "blood necklaces."
> • I sewed myself an amulet for my altar: a leather bag containing a piece of material with the menstrual blood of an important friend, a dried rose hip, a dried rose bud, and a dried chili pepper. Red Hot!
> • At the moment, I'm sewing together a cloak using only red, pink, yellow, and orange cloth rags, or cloth printed with red, pink, or yellow flowers. (I can't sew well, so it'll be a while before I can throw it around me and withdraw into my lair.)

Special menstrual clothing, jewelry, and amulets make the charged, changed condition of menstruation very obvious and help you focus your dragontime energy. As soon as you put on your amulet, you enter into another time, another plane, into a magical world where you meet other forces and experiences. Special objects work as keys to connect to certain powers.

> • Blood helps the shaman enter into her special world.
> • Amulets of fur and feathers impart strong animal-totem energy.
> • Dream pillows can connect you to plants.

In Africa I've seen clay altar figures, red on the belly and black on back. They're made in the form of animals, or many-breasted women, or human figures without sexual organs. The dark back is said to radiate power, to be strong and protective. The red front side is said to be soft, open, and warm. In the case of danger, the figure is set in the window or the door, black side facing outwards. When companionship is sought, the figure is placed with the red side facing out.

Power Objects

On your altar or used in rituals, power objects can connect you to other women, ancient and modern, who have bled and bleed now; they can help you connect to the power of your own bleeding.

• **Bowl-shaped stones, and stone pestles** are prehistoric tools closely tied to menstruation and fertility. Bowls held blood and grain, milk and honey. They held gifts for the ancestors and ancient spirits. Pestles, besides grinding grain and herbs, could, if small enough, be held in the vagina to relieve cramps, increase fertility, or simply arouse passion.

• **Cauldrons and gourd vessels** remind us of the belly of women and the power of the uterus (creation). Everything is "cooked" inside it—in other words, discussed, woven, enchanted—whatever needs to be done. (See Cauldron pgs. 23-27.)

• **Drums** give us rhythms that move body and soul, carrying us into wonderful trance states. Try dancing to a strong drum beat to release menstrual cramps and tension. The farther apart your legs and the deeper you bend your knees, the more your belly will relax.

• **Feathers** remind us of the flight of the soul, the ability to leave one's body, visions, trance journeys, dream images, and spiritual contact with the ancestresses. [Bead or wrap the feather shaft to maintain its energy.]

• **Menstrual blood** is protective magic and strong energy. Use it to protect your daughter or your doorway against unwelcome visitors. Use it to seal spells and strengthen decisions. Use it on cloth, stone, or paper. You can even paint yourself with your menstrual blood. [From a discreet daub in the middle of the forehead to thighs streaked with crimson. And, oh, those rosy cheeks!]

• **Meteorite** stones bring power from other worlds and the power of the underworld. They can help you refine your perceptions and decipher vibrations.

• **Mud, clay, soil, and earth** enable us to make visible whatever we have magically envisioned. Form clay into little menstrual dolls, goddesses, and vessels. Make beads for a power necklace in the form of tiny animals and figures. [Plant seeds; get your hands dirty.]

• **Opals** are said to have magic powers, to contain secrets. Lyrical descriptions of opal comment on its dark, deep power which endangers those who don't know how to work with it. For me, the opal is a true magic stone, one in close relationship with the unique energy of menstruation. And, yes, this energy pulls you down into the depths.

• **Red stones** are menstrual blood in rock form. Sacred ochre, hematite (blood stone), and all other high iron content rocks are deemed especially magical by primitive people. (Red rocks are rich in iron.) Some of these make a red powder when ground. [And this powder is widely used to "decorate" homes, tombs, women.] Other good menstrual stones include carnelian, red coral, rubies, garnets, red quartz, and amber, too. To even out irregular, unpleasant periods, wear these stones as necklaces. To help relieve menstrual pain, lay them in the vagina (which is a lot of fun).

• **Sea shells** evoke the ocean, la mer, Mary, the female gender. Sea shells have been used by women of almost every culture to increase passion, fertility, and hearty enjoyment of the belly's power. (Cowrie shells are especially valued.)

• **Wool yarn** in *red and yellow* colors is wrapped around an object or braided together to solidify menstrual magic. The special powers of your bleeding time can be used to bind and release. And everything that is bound must sometime be released.

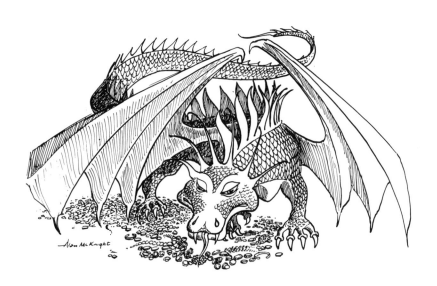

Moon and Blood

There is hardly a [modern white] woman who can say, "When I bleed on the new moon, full moon, or waxing quarter, then I feel so and so." So few of us are aware of the phases of the moon or how it affects our menses. When we do notice, it's when the full moon and menstruation happen at the same time. This is experienced as especially dramatic, or wonderful, or painful, or special in some other way.

The natural cycle of women who live and sleep out in the open away from artificial light is to ovulate on the full moon and menstruate on the new moon. The Taureg women I visit in Africa concur with this. For women of the neon civilization, though, it's almost impossible to follow this moon/menstrual cycle (although it would probably bring about the easiest menstruations, for, as already said, full moon and menstruation at the same time can be an overwhelming experience).

In 1979, an excellently researched special issue of *Courage* dealt specifically with menstrual blood. In it Louise Lacey, author of *Lunaceptions* tells how she regulated her ovulation by sleeping three nights out of twenty-nine in light and the others in pitch black.

My observations of the effect of moon phases on menstruation are compiled from the experiences of women I've lived with, worked with, done workshops with, met over the course of years, or just talked to casually about their bleeding.

When moon phase energies are noticed, and these energies magnified by menstruation, what specific powers can be freed up and made available for use? *Can be.* I do not say that it must be so, or should be so, or that you will experience it so. Only that it is possible, if you want to work with it.

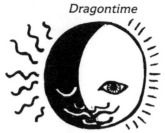

Waxing Moon Menstruation

Waxing moon is growth, time to learn, listen, and feel. New processes are coming into play, new experiences and events are within reach. Dawn reddens the sky, day begins, air moves, the moon is waxing.

The energy of waxing moon menstruation is inwards, self-nourishing. It's time to think, to learn, to read. Time to make new discoveries. During this time, you might be open to important learning, and to receiving knowledge from other women.

The animal of the waxing moon menstruation is the raven, who stands for the transference of knowledge and embodies the flight of the soul. Persephone, the goddess who walked the path to the underworld and was initiated into womanly bleeding, is the guardian of this menstrual phase.

Full Moon Menstruation

The full moon is vitality: time to work changes, to make decisions, to show one's power, to bring something into being, to work politically. Noontime heat spreads in waves across the sky, fiery energy at its peak, streaming power evoking earthly blooms.

The energy of full moon menstruation is outward, world-nourishing. You have to be a real bundle of energy to be happy and satisfied with your work under this charged condition. Feasts and celebrations go well with full moon bleeding. During this time, the most powerful magic can be worked and influence exerted. The volcano already pours forth; the fire need only be controlled and directed. Now is the time to learn to transform energy: turn rage into creative action, belly cramps into sensuousness.

The animal of the full moon menstruation is the Phoenix, mythical bird being, who burns to ashes in order to rise anew. Ishtar, the Red Goddess of Babylon is the guardian of this menstrual fire.

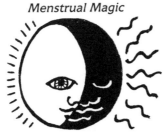

Waning Moon Menstruation

The waning moon is a fire that has dwindled, having already given some of its heat to nourish others. Now is the time for persistence, for making reality out of the visions and impulses. The sun sets, darkness settles, the sky fills with the light of countless universes. The moon is waning.

The energy of waning moon bleeding is outward, world-nourishing. It's the time to tend the blooms of the full moon energy, to create in the world what you have already created in your imagination. Weave your web: substantiate discoveries, verify knowledge, develop your plans and projects, stabilize already existing conditions.

The animal of this waning moon menstruation is the she-bear, who, in old myths is the womb. The energy of the bear is mighty, deep, motherly. The goddess of this time, Demeter, is responsible for the cycles of life on earth, letting the fruits and grains ripen for harvest, in preparation for the next cycle when she'll withdraw to tend to her own nourishment, letting the earth become barren while she mourns her daughter.

New Moon Menstruation

The new moon is the hidden moon, the dark and mysterious power of the deep. The new moon is the pull inwards. The void sucks energy in and, at the same time, gives all power. During this time, anxieties, memories, and experiences may rise up, eager to be dealt with. Midnight: darkness at it fullest, a velvet ocean, watery womb of all life, the moon is new. The moon breathes in; the belly breathes out.

The energy of new moon bleeding is inwards, self-nourishing, into the cauldron of the woman, the belly, the witches' cauldron, the holy grail. New moon menstruation is a strong time of healing and its element is water. It's a good time to take stock, to read old diaries, to look through old photo albums, and to draw conclusions from them. What is built up on the full moon is dissolved on the new moon; that includes binding and releasing spells.

The animal of the new moon menstruation is the toad, with all her knowledge, her slipperiness, her ability to be quite alone, and her untouchable (poisonous) exterior. The goddess of this time is Hecate, the woman at the joining of three roads [also called tri-via], the guardian of mysteries and knowledge, the reaper, the dark one, the crone.

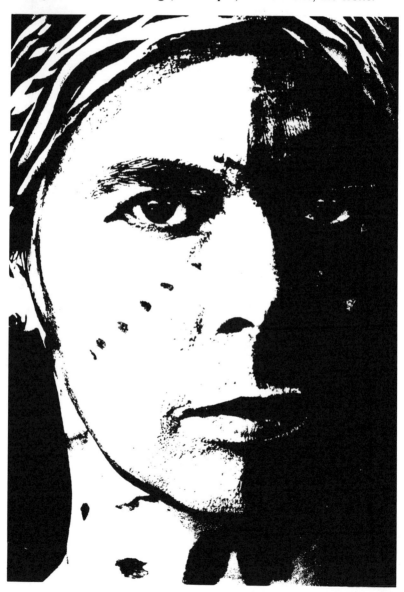

Dragontime Allies

As teachers of truth, as oracles, and as priceless treasures, the animals and plants of our world ally themselves with us. A dictionary of allies, archetypes, and power places especially connected to menstrual magic follows.

Animal Allies

(Goddess names added by Susun.)

• **Bears, especially she-bears,** are the womb, the belly, knowledge of the energies of the menstrual cycle [herbal wisdom]. Ursi, Ursula, Artio.

• **Bees** are matriarchy (the queen bee!), the earth's abundance and fertility, nourishment, sweetness. (In some stories, women change to honey bees or bumblebees and swarm out at night. Woe if their window should be shut; unable to get back in, they die.) Demeter, Deborah, Melissa.

• **Birds** are the flight of the soul, ancestral spirits. Ba, Angel, Maat, Krake. See also *Owls*.

• **Cats** are knowledge of the earth's ley (energy) lines and water veins, the seventh sense [many lives, matrifocal culture, solar wisdom.] Bast, Sekmet, Freya, Cybele.

• **Cows** are the patient wisdom of old, matrilinear cultures, abundance, sensual life force, bodily strength. [Holy cow!] Hathor, Bo, Audumla, Io, Europa.

During my pregnancy many years ago, and later too, when I menstruated, I often experienced a strong craving for raw flesh. I would eat it, with a little lemon, while I was still out on the street. Finally, I ritualized this strange habit, and called on the animal whose flesh I ate raw—the cow. A very intense experience with Hathor, the cow goddess of Egypt, followed. Since then, my meat hunger is much less. I acknowledge this lustful, cannibalistic feeling, the desire to have something "bloody," even though it repulses me at the same time.

• **Hares** are fertility, the power of night, shape shifting. (In a number of myths, menstruating women change themselves into hares and fly to the moon at night.) Eoster.

• **Owls** are wisdom, knowledge of the night, ability to move about in darkness, precision, invisibility. Athena, Lilith, Minerva, Anath.

• **Snakes** are sexual energy, immortality, divination, death and rebirth (they shed their skins), menstruation. Kundalini, Nehushtah, UaZit, Buto.

• **Spiders** are dream weaving, spinning, magic, measuring, networking, being wrapped up in yourself. Arachne, Sussistanako, Anansi (Aunt Nancy).

• **Toads and frogs** are fertility, warmth, the moist slippery belly, spreading out. [Totem of the pregnant/birthing woman, the womb of regeneration.) Bufo.

• **Wolves** are watchfulness, austerity, shamanic knowledge, connections to other worlds [singer, pathfinder]. Artemis, Lupus, Feronia.

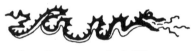

Archetypal Allies

• **Air** carries dreams and stories and scents. You can ride the air at dragontime. Your sense of smell is particularly keen during dragontime. Don't suffer cramped muscles from oxygen depletion during your menstruation. Use aromatic herbs and fragrant oils in your menstrual hut (an oil diffuser will help carry the scent through the air) to change your mood and remind you to breathe deeply. (See Green Allies, pages 67-71.) If you fear cramps or pain (back pain as well) and the fear prevents you from breathing deeply, you've unconsciously intensified the problem, as oxygen starved muscles cramp more easily.

• **Bear Mother** gives advice in all problems of mother's and women's bodies. You can see her in the sky as the Big Dipper.

• **Dragon woman** holds undomesticated wilderness, the original condition of the world. She is communication through all pores, a fire spitter [and a treasure guarder].

• **Earth** is our mother. Mossy soil absorbs your bleeding. In summer, it's wonderful to bleed into the earth. Stamping and dancing connects you to earthy powers during your bleeding time.

• **Fire** is the dragon's power. Menstrual blood is fiery water. You can symbolically take on the power of fire by jumping over it, or burning something in the fire. Fire is warmth as well. Bring her to your dragontime with hot water bottles, warm blankets, warm socks, and tender communication.

• **Habergeiss** helps you change. Traditionally, a kind of she-devil that appears as a ghost. She stands for the power of ancient matrifocal religions, and for nonconformity. She's a shrewd, crafty, and ironic observer. She urges you to step over the edge.

• **Lilith** is the goddess who "couples with demons" and bears a hundred children every day. She refused to be Adam's subservient wife, preferring her own domain, and repulsed three angels sent to fetch her back after she left Adam. The *lilim* are her daughters; they are women expert at love-making and filled with lust; also known as succubi.

• **Madame Death** (in Bohemia, Death Woman) shows you how to change forms. The dark crone comes when it's time to leave outmoded ways. Sit with her in pear trees (in Austria) and in apple trees (in Czechoslovakia.) The crone or grandmother is the ancient woman of the crossroads who tests you and may give you great treasures. [She calls upon your patience.]

• **Mermaid** draws you into the deep, teaching you to let go.

• **Phoenix** reminds the menstruating woman that being consumed by fire can renew her. For instance, don't avoid pain and cramps. Go into them, dance into them, scream them aloud, burn them, entrust them to Phoenix, and receive new power.

• **Sphinx** is a Goddess of death and rebirth, lion-headed, fierce. Another form of "she who bleeds and does not die."

• **Trickster** [Coyote/Raccoon/Fool] puts you to the test; brings confusion and chaos. Try eating cherries with this one.

• **Water** moves and flows. Take on the power of water by bathing, by releasing (cry, laugh), and by allowing your menstrual blood to flow. Water is our first home. Bring her to your bleeding in the form of warm soups and herbal teas.

• **Weavers** are those who weave the threads of the world. They can cast spells and bring about the impossible. They will help you out if you're in need, but, in thanks, you must invite them to dinner. When questioned, one must never deny one's connection to them, even if they're shapeless and repulsive. They usually reside in caves.

• **Whore/Bad Girl/Red Witch** [reawakens the magical powers of your self-centered sexuality. She helps you to touch with true intimacy and to experience ecstasy in everyday acts.]

• **Woods-woman/Wildwoman/Green Witch** connects you to nature, to the knowledge of healing plants and nature magic.

[See "Tales of the Cairds" by Anne Cameron for an excellent and extensive dictionary of "the magic ones"—from Baniks and Brownies to Pixies and Trolls.]

 **Power Places**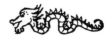

• **Caves** are the womb of the goddess as well as the womb of the earth. Nowhere else are you closer to your own female power. Caves are good places to meditate and seek visions. Be sure beforehand that you can find the way out and that you'll be safe in the cave. I never go alone into an unknown cave.

The caves of my Middle European mountains were almost all ritual sites during the Stone Age. Special finds have been made in the Altmuhl Valley, the Schwaben Alps, the Hagen mountains, and in the Dolomites and Toten mountains. A good hiking guide will mention monuments and ritual sites near you.

[Caves are traditionally places of safety, connection, marriage, treasure, and magical birth.]

• **Crossroads** (the junction of roads) are places of strong energy, intensified where three roads come together, and where oaks grow. Some have the power to dissolve depression and anxiety. Set yourself in the middle and feel the different possible paths. Decisions can be made at crossroads. [Crossroads are dedicated to Trivia; she of three (tri) ways (via).]

• **Groves** of trees are the most ancient sites of goddess worship. In a grove you experience deep peace and spiritual power. Where whole groves of the same kind of tree grow, the energies are exceptionally powerful. The Celts favored oak groves for their rituals. In Mesopotamia and Sumer, acacia, cedar, or cypress groves were preferred. At Starnberg Lake, there's a grove (perhaps the last in Germany) entirely of yews. Near home, I go to an old beech grove. [Grove Goddesses include Diana, Nemesis, Silvania, and Asherah.]

• **Mounds** also called "fairy mounds" or grave mounds, are set into the landscape like pregnant bellies or full breasts and so by association are regarded as places of life and death. (Long ago, the dead were buried in a fetal position to show that death and new life are the same.) Mounds are powerful places for dancing and ritualizing.

• **Springs** are my favorite power places. Since the time of the Celts, the springs of the British Isles have been sacred Goddess shrines.

[Springs are the source. They give life, purity, and continuous refreshment. Hot springs, especially in western North America, have been spiritual/ritual sites for time out of mind.]

Many springs bear goddess names such as Brigid or Mary. Springs are places where nymphs reside. Always, springs have been places of pilgrimage; Catholics and Pagans alike, all seek the healing waters. Springs teach us to let go, to relax and to be moved by the flow of change.

• **Stone** (or **megalithic** from "great stone") **circles** are prehistoric ritual sites. They are always located on earth energy centers and ley lines (energy lines). (Stone circles apparently amplify the ley lines.)

Cornwall, England, has many stone circles known by maidens' and women's names. At a certain stone circle in Southern Cornwall, witches are said to meet; traces of parties and meetings are certainly to be seen aplenty. In stone circles, I recharge myself, find new energy, and dip into ancient memories.

• **"Witching" places/dance sites** are everywhere. Mountain caves, groves of trees, meadows, clearings, plateaus, and cliffs named "Witch" or "Dance" something are common throughout Europe. I believe this indicates these places were ancient ceremonial sites especially sacred to women, perhaps even menstrual ritual sites. [In North America, similar sites may be found. They are sometimes known as "birthing circles." In a public park in Ann Arbor, Michigan, I found myself in an oval clearing surrounded by red trillium, wild ginger, life root, and other plants especially useful for women's problems; obviously, from the look and feel, an ancient (and much used) menstrual ritual site. In Ontario, local land holders showed me to another ancient site, now thickly guarded by poison ivy and raspberry thorns.] I dance, cast spells, and dream in these places. They strengthen the power of the uterus and awaken the inner wisdom.

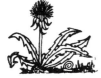

Green Allies

• **Apple** (*Malus species*) is the fruit of the Goddess, symbolizing her life force and joyousness. Apples sometimes represent the menstruating woman as well. [Did Eve actually eat an apple? Unlikely. She was Mediterranean; apples aren't.]

• **Basil** (*Ocimum basilicum*) oil or fresh leaf tea stimulates bleeding, awakens the life force, and chases off feelings of helplessness. The aroma is quite strong; I like it with camphor or juniper. [My favorite way to "take" basil is as pesto! Combine 1 cup/250 ml. olive oil, same amount fresh basil, several cloves garlic, some pine nuts or walnuts (not much), and a spoonful of Parmesan cheese in your blender. Whir. Serve over warm noodles or vegetables. Wow!]

• **Benzoin** (*Styrax benzoin*) is extracted from the root of a desert tree. The odor brings sunshine, cheer and warmth into the belly, though some find it offensively aromatic.

• **Bloodroot** (*Sanguinaria canadensis*) [is not to be used internally. Yes, the roots bleed when you break them. For dragontime rituals and altars, bloodroot (roots, of course) offer wisdom about release and bringing on the red flow.]

• **Camphor** (*Cinnamomum camphora*) oil is anti-depressant. It helps you breathe deeply. [Caution: Don't use essential oils internally. Even the smell of, or skin contact with, some essential oils may cause an allergic reaction.]

• **Catnip** (*Nepeta cataria*) [fresh leaves make a tea treasured by dragon mothers. Pain-killing, cramp-easing, and belly-soothing, calming catnip tea is an ally for bleeding women and crying babies.]

• **Chamomile** (*Chamaelum nobile* and *Matricaria recutita*) oil or flower tea calms. Especially as a steam in a room, or as a warm tea, chamomile soothes the nerves and gives a feeling of peaceful warmth.

• **Cinnamon** (*Cinnamomum* zeylanicum) sticks or oil make the soul warm and awaken the feeling of security. It's very pungent and reminds me pleasantly of Christmas. [To slow profuse bleeding, try hot apple cider/juice with lots of cinnamon.]

• **Cronewort/Mugwort** (*Artemisia vulgaris*) [is the herb of Artemis, wild virgin, moon goddess, woman-lover, healer, herbalist, midwife. Use dried leaves and flowers of Cronewort in your dragon lair as a smudge, for dream pillows, and in vision amulets. Cronewort offers you stories, guidance, and deep slumber with vivid, colorful dreams. She is the one-who-keeps-her-wise-blood-inside, the crone who is also the virgin.] In German, also known as woman's weed, or power herb.

• **Elder** (*Sambucus species*) has long been synonymous with the power to heal, the wisdom of the ancestresses, and the presence of ancient goddesses. [Elda Mor, the wise old woman in the elder, gives me elder-berries to use as body-paint as well as for jam and wine. She gives me flowers for my altar, ah! I made a magic wand from the branch she broke into my hand . . . tinctured by full moon light, her lacy flowers soothe the children's fevers.]

• **Eucalyptus** (*Eucalyptus species*) oil or leaf tea gives a clear, un-quenchable energy. Shakes loose rigid patterns. Very strong. Recom-mended only for robust women wishing to refresh themselves.

• **Ginger** (*Zingiber officinalis*) [spreads warmth, moves energy, eases cramps, brings on the flow (not an abortifacient), soothes the belly, disperses gas, and calms a queasy stomach. She's an important dragon-time ally.]

• **Honey** is sacred food, teaching us softness and patience.

• **Hyssop** (*Hyssopus officinalis*) leaf tea or oil strengthens and cheers. In addition, this almost forgotten herb is a disinfectant. [Some women dislike the smell very much.]

• **Juniper** or **cedar** (*Juniperus species*) oil or smoke from burning dried needles rebuilds the fibers of the aura, heals the invisible layers, and helps soothe women who are bleeding very heavily.

• **Ladies Mantle** (*Alchemilla vulgaris*) leaf and flower tea, brings on the flow of blood, helps you let go, dissolves.

• **Lavender** (*Lavendula species*) oil or flower tea stimulates bleeding in women who have scanty or irregular menses. A favorite scent for dream-ing and storytelling. [Use the flowers in dream/vision pillows, on your altar, and throughout your menstrual hut.]

• **Lemon balm** (*Melissa officinalis*) oil or leaf tea awakens fantasy and dreams. Resonates to the same harmony as the belly. A little lemon balm oil mixed with a few drops of lavender and orange oil and put in a few ounces of olive or almond oil can be used as a massage oil to induce trance states.

• **Life root** (*Senecio aureus*) [has allied bleeding and birthing women for hundreds of thousands of years. Her flowers were found carefully placed in the oldest grave yet known. I tincture the blossoms in late May, then use 5-10 drops daily to help regulate menstrual cycling, ease pre-menstrual problems, and relieve even severe menstrual distress (vomiting and intense cramps). Best results occur with long-term use (several months at least), rather than acute intervention. Although many *Senecios* are poisonous, the three species used in Europe and North America—*aureus, jacobea,* and *vulgaris*—have extensive folkloric validations of safety and effectiveness. Doses of 15-25 drops may be used to facilitate a "stuck" or stalled labor, repeated 2-3 times per hour for up to two hours.]

• **Lipped flowers**, for instance snapdragons, orchids, and mint blossoms evoke the vagina and women's sexual energy. [On the menstrual altar, they bring the magic of enclosing, taking in.]

• **Mandrake** (*Mandragora officinatum*) is a root thought to possess many magical powers, some associated with menstruation. In German, she is called "Dragon Spice."

• **Millet** (*Eleusine coracana*) grain is a sacred food of the ancients, a wisdom bringer. She quiets the mind and helps relieve cramps. [Add ½ cup/125 ml. millet grain to 1 cup/250 ml. boiling water. Cover and reduce heat. Simmer for 15-25 minutes, until dry and tender. For a softer grain, use more water.]

• **Motherwort** (*Leonurus cardiaca*) [has sharp seed pods used ritually to draw away pain during childbirth and menstruation. Her fresh flowers and leaves make a tincture wonderfully calming (10 drops), easing to menstrual pain (15 drops), and relieving to hot flashes (20 drops). She is a most important Dragontime ally.]

• **Mugwort** (see *Cronewort*)

• **Nettle** (*Urtica dioica*) [leaf infusion strengthens the kidneys and adrenals and helps you get rid of excess water. A nourisher beyond compare, Nettle is rich in iron, calcium, vitamin K, carotenes, and protein. She is an especially beneficial ally for women who bleed heavily.]

• **Orange** (*Citrus species*) blossom oil or tea smells like an excursion of the soul to the sun. Reminds me of childhood and security. Not overly aromatic, but very healing, bringing ease, even bliss.

• **Peppermint** (*Mentha piperita*) oil or leaf tea lets the spirit rise up. (In the African desert, peppermint infusion is prepared so strong that one hallucinates after consuming it.) The smell of peppermint strengthens bleeding and stimulates the flow. [In infusion with yarrow, mint is a powerful emmenagogue and diuretic.]

• **Pomegranate** (*Punica granafum*) fruit has been, since ancient times, a symbol of woman's sexuality and menstrual blood, of the womb and the vagina. The many depictions of pomegranates throughout history show, in context, the power of women. Since the Inquisition, pomegranates have disappeared almost completely from the visual symbolism of our culture.

• **Pumpkin** (*Curcurbita pepo*) seeds make everything flow. Fertility and abundance are yours when you ally with pumpkins, gourds, and watermelons.

• **Raspberry** (*Rubus species*) leaves and stalks represent woman's passion and life force. The tea brings happiness and passionate menstruation. [Brambles such as raspberry heal the earth, evoking friendship and sisterhood. A raspberry leaf infusion eases pre-menstrual tension and menstrual cramps while tonifying and strengthening the womb.]

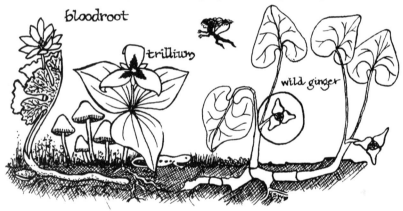

• **Red trillium** (*Trillium Species*) [displays three-part leaves and three-part red flowers to announce her strong female medicine. Enjoy looking; don't pick her. Symbolizing completion, and sisterhood, used by midwives and spirit healers, trilliums have led me to Native American menstrual ritual sites.]

• **Red Clover** (*Trifolium pratense*) blossoms, filled with buzzing honey bees, evoke the power of the Red Goddess of Babylon or Sawuska, and the poetry of Sappho. [Red clover infusion can increase fertility, encourage menstrual regularity, and ease mood swings.]

• **Rose** (*Rosa species*) oil and fresh blossoms, though usually outrageously, unreachably expensive, give me a feeling of harmony. The thorns protect the rose and your womb/belly. The smell of rose oil stimulates the flow of blood. Rosehips, a sacred fruit in ancient times, evoke pleasure, happiness, and red-smeared lips. Roses are relaxing.

• **Rosemary** (*Rosmarinus officinalis*) leaf tea strengthens the body and spirit, stimulates bleeding, helps you be alert and happy, and stabilizes the spirit when it's too light and tends to float away. The oil is middle intensity, strong but not pushy. The smell of rosemary chases away nausea. [Rosemary symbolizes the power of woman as family leader. She evokes clarity.]

• **Sage** (*Salvia officinalis*) oil or leaf steadies the mind and the flow. The smell of the burning plant is very evocative. [Sage tea reduces or stops a heavy flow.]

• **Thyme** (*Thymus species*) oil or fresh leaves have a sharp odor, astringent and antiseptic. Let this scent help you when you're totally exhausted and over the edge, when you need to withdraw into yourself and be by yourself.

• **Watermelon**: *(See Pumpkin)*

• **Wild ginger** (*Asarum canadensis*) [with its pelvic-shaped leaves and dark red uterus-like flowers is used symbolically and as a tea or tincture (of the roots) for warming and strengthening the belly.]

• **Yarrow** (*Achillea millefolium*) flowers, leaves, and stalks, hold the knowledge of the ancestresses. [Yarrow is used worldwide as an oracular ally. From casting the I Ching with yarrow stalks to sleeping with a yarrow flower pillow . . . awaiting a dream of the beloved, this graceful, amazingly aromatic herb has a long history as Dragontime ally. A strong tea will bring on your bloods (not an abortifacient), nourish your nerves, and help you eliminate excess water.]

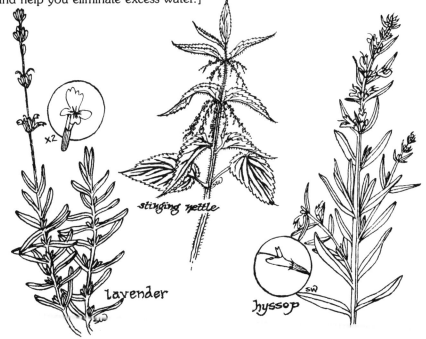

x2

stinging nettle

lavender

hyssop

Dragon-Day Brews

[Infusions are generally preferable to teas; they contain greater quantities of vitamins, minerals, proteins, and medicinal components such as alkaloids. Feel free to season your infusions with honey, sugar, milk, tamari, or to dilute them. Except when noted, up to a quart a day can be consumed.

[Steep a teaspoon/1-2 grams of dried herb for 5-10 minutes in a cup/250 ml. of hot water for a **tea**. Steep one ounce/28 grams of dried herb for 4-8 hours in a quart/liter jar filled with boiling water and capped for an **infusion**.]

• **Tasty tea for Dragontime:** 1 ounce/28 grams each nettle (*Urtica*) and raspberry (*Rubus*) leaves, a pinch of mugwort (*Artemisia vulgaris*) and a few fennel (*Foeniculum vulgare*) seeds; use a teaspoonful to the cup.
• **Tea to help women with heavy bleeding and cramps:** equal parts horsetail (*Equisetum*), catnip (*Nepeta cataria*), and shepherd's purse (*Capsella bursa-pastoris*). [Best if fresh herbs are used in this particular brew, as dried catnip and shepherd's purse are often without value.]
• **Refreshing, healing tea for dragontime women and crones:** equal parts dulse seaweed and lemon balm (*Melissa*). Yum!
• **Infusion to help women with menstrual pain and tension:** in a quart/liter of boiling water steep one-third ounce (10 grams) each strawberry leaves (*Fragaria*), raspberry leaves (*Rubus*), and comfrey leaves (*Symphytum*).
• **Infusion to help nourish you during menstruation:** steep an ounce/30 grams of stinging nettle (*Urtica*) in a quart/liter of water. You may wish to add a hint of mugwort/cronewort (*Artemisia vulgaris*).
• **Infusion to calm and nourish young women just starting menstruation:** one-half ounce (15 grams) comfrey (*Symphytum*) leaves plus an inch of licorice (*Glycyrrhiza glabra*) root or dong quai (*Angelica sinensis*) root brewed overnight in one quart/liter of water.
• **Infusion to bring on a missed period:** one-third ounce/10 grams each of rosemary *(Rosmarinus off.)*, parsley *(Petroselinum crispus)*, and roman chamomile *(Chamaelum nobile)* plus a pinch of yew *(Taxas canadensis)* bark in a quart/liter of water. [Note that yew is considered poisonous.]
• **Infusion to help prevent osteoporosis after menopause:** to a quart/liter of water, one ounce/28 grams nettle (*Urtica dioica*) and a large pinch of horsetail (*Equisetum arvense*). Two cups daily is a good amount.

Dragontime Trance Journeys

Whether or not you have an actual menstrual hut, you always have your own interior dragon lair, where you can withdraw to be quiet and heal yourself. Many women feel especially vulnerable during menstruation and are empowered by trance journeys to fantasy places where they feel well, happy, and secure. Many women find their intuitive abilities are stronger during their period. Perhaps you'll find it easier then too, to have out-of-body experiences, to let your spirit fly, and to come in contact with the ancient ones and the old mythical beings such as dragons.

[Trance journeys are different from, but also called, guided visualizations, creative imagining, daydreams, focused fantasy, and self-hypnosis.]

With practice, you'll come to know your own inner spaces and you'll create your own trance journeys, but, to start you off, I'll give you a wonderful basic relaxation and five of my favorite trance journeys.

Before every trance journey I do a focused relaxation. I find physical and mental relaxation prerequisite to imaginative/spiritual agility, whether for storytelling, dreaming, or journeying. Children go on magical voyages when they're required to nap and aren't sleepy. When you have a fever and must be idle, does your spirit begin to adventure, to explore, to journey?

Before your relaxation and trance journey, air out the room where you'll be. Burn some aromatic herbs, or incense, or put some fragrant oil in the oil diffuser. Unplug the phone, block the door bell, and hang a sign on the door, "Do not disturb. I'm dreaming." Or like my daughter Walli: "Danger. Do not Enter. Dragon at home." Allow this peacefulness to affect you. Give yourself time to feel your way into your space, to relax, and to become surrounded by your own good energy.

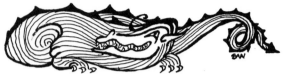

Dragontime Relaxation

Feel your body. Say to every part of your body, "You are totally relaxed and loose." Start with the toes, then move to the soles of your feet . . . then the ankles . . . calves . . . knees . . . thighs . . . buttocks . . . vagina . . . uterus . . . all the inner organs . . . belly . . . breasts . . . fingers . . . hands . . . arms . . . elbows . . . upper arms . . . shoulders . . . throat . . . neck . . . spine . . . all the back muscles . . . jaw . . . ears . . . scalp . . . mouth . . . tongue . . . forehead . . . brain . . . and skull. Name, step by step each part of your body and say, "My feet (or whatever) are relaxed and loose." Someone can recite for you or you can do it yourself. Here's the relaxing rhyme of my friend Wilfriede: "Your foot relaxes to the core, now you feel it no more."

As you relax, focus on your breath. Let it flow calmly through your relaxed body. Breathe in; a tingling sensation goes through all your cells as they are showered with oxygen. Breathe out; feel relaxation spread through your muscles, nerves and bone.

Breathe in and out calmly until your mind and body are very quiet.

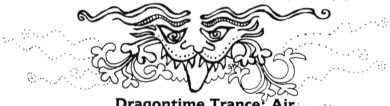

Dragontime Trance: Air

Relax. Allow yourself to envision or imagine that you're lying on a cloud. Feel its softness and gentleness. You lie as though on cottonballs floating through the air. The cloud sweeps over a summer field. Try to recognize the separate smells: pine, wild herbs, flowers, cow dung, hay (no one has hay fever in a trance, so enjoy).

Slowly the cloud carries you out to sea. Smell the tangy, sharp odor of the ocean, hear the screaming of the seagulls. As you blow over the open sea, the wind rocks you, making a strange music on the water, whistling and humming.

Now direct the cloud to places you especially love. Look at them from above. You may imagine that a bird accompanies you, sitting beside you. Let it take you on its back for closer looks, if you wish.

When you're finished, return gently to your body. Imagine first the humming of many voices, or bees, or the strings of a harp played by the wind. (Wind-harp sounds are truly magical.) Then come back into your body by moving your toes, feet and legs, fingers, hands and arms. Stretch and yawn, make faces, lay your hands on your belly. Give yourself a short time to think back over the trip. [Then write it down, draw a picture of it, sing it, or tell it as a story.]

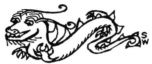

Dragontime Trance: Earth

Relax. Allow yourself to envision or imagine that you're on a path winding through a landscape. You're creating this landscape. [Is it rocky? wooded? filled with wildflowers? summer? winter? day? night?] It is just as you want it.

Suddenly your road takes off in a steep incline and goes down a hill to a gully. In front of you a cliff rises. In the middle of the cliff is a cave. You climb up into the opening of the cave. After quite a narrow entrance, there's a biggish underground room. Perhaps it's not quite dark because some light is coming through a hole in the rock wall. Perhaps the room is totally dark. [Even in the dark, you can see.]

Look at the walls of the cave. What do you see? Are there jewels there? Onyx? Opals? Garnets or rubies? Crystals?

Walk or move around the cave as you need to. What else is there?

This is your menstrual cave, this is your dragon lair. Everything is here that you need at any moment. Any food and drink you can imagine is here. Your allies will come here: plant helpers, goddesses, animal totems; anyone you wish can join you here. Call them, if you'd like, or wait to see who visits you. Notice every detail; in such a way you'll discover your secret wishes and needs.

In my menstrual cave I can allow myself everything that eludes me in reality. I dissolve; I step over the edge with my senses; I learn, look, smell, and eat whatever I want. Visitors come often. Some are greeted with pleasure. Those I don't want are brusquely thrown out. Sometimes, ancestresses come and tell me stories, a wonderful experience. In the realm of your trance, *you* alone are the boss, and no one can overrule you.

When you leave your cave, depart with the knowledge that you can return at any time. Don't cling to anything, but do write everything down afterwards.

Return to your body gently, as described in the air trance.

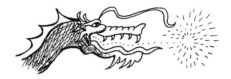

Dragontime Trance: Fire

Light a candle or sit by a fire. Relax.

Your path into the fire is known to the dragon crone who lives on the other side of the river at the end of the world, between heaven and earth.

Commence with an image of a boat, riding on the river at the end of the world. The river is gray. It has no beginning, no end, no shore. There are no fish and no birds. Crags rise in the distance: three pyramid-shaped crags. Behind them smoke curls into the air.

After a long ride, you climb out of the boat and step onto dry land. What is it like? How do the crags look now? What do you feel? Is it warm or cold? What do you smell?

You walk around the crags. There stands an ancient woman. She's stirring a cauldron. What does she look like? How is she dressed? Is she human? Half human, half animal? Look at her closely.

Then look at the cauldron. What is the cauldron like? What's in it? What's cooking there? What do you want to cook there? It stands over a fire which is being blown from the nostrils of a little dragon. [Look deeply into the fire.] What do you want to burn or transform in the fire? [Speak to the crone or the dragon if you wish. Stare into the fire. What do you see?]

When you're done perhaps you'll fly back on the dragon! Remember that this fire where you can find advice and help and transformation is always accessible to you.

Return to your body gently as in the air trance.

In connection with fire, the Inquisition (witch-burning) fires, deserve mention. It may be important to you to experience death by fire in a trance journey sometime. (Hopefully you'll have the skillful guidance of someone you trust). But remember, not all women were witches (or priestesses, queens, healers) in a past life.

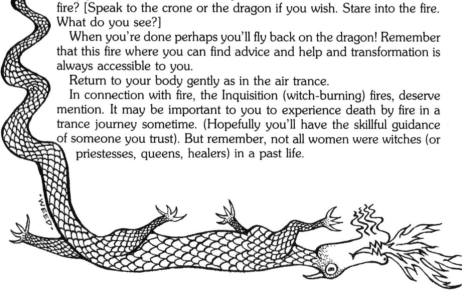

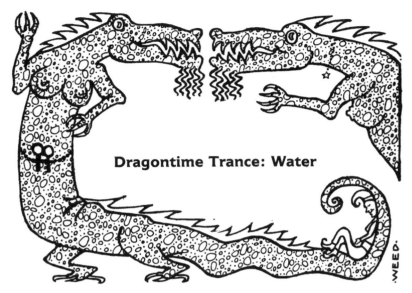

Dragontime Trance: Water

Think about water for a while. [Play koto, harp, or other "watery" music.] Diffuse lavender (or your favorite oil) into the air.

Does water mean "to be drowned in tears?" Did you wet your bed as a child? Does sweating bother you? Give yourself permission to feel your own liquidness. Everything you are is in flow. Feel your way into your pulsing bodily fluids as you relax.

Relax even more deeply. Now envision or imagine that you are being blown, light as a feather, over the surface of the water. When you're ready, dive down, down into the depths of the ocean. Perhaps you'd like to change into a seal, or a whale, or a dolphin?

Look at the colors; observe the fishes. You have no enemies in this water. Everyone knows you're coming to heal yourself, and feels friendly toward you. The sharks grin at you. Dive down as deep as you want.

Now imagine a gigantic, iridescent shell. Look at it and feel it carefully, noting its colors and shape. Curl up inside the shell, if you wish. Listen to how it whooshes and hums, echoing the ocean's song. What do you feel like in this shell under the sea?

Seek out a meeting with the beings of the deep. Let pictures rise up like bubbles in water. What do they show you? Who visits you in your shell?

When you've had enough, swim up high again, or let yourself be carried by a fish or a dolphin. Return to yourself gently as before, remembering to make some record of your adventures.

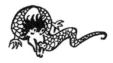

Dragontime Trance: Journey into the Womb

This journey helps women experience dragontime from the inside out. If your belly is swollen pre-menstrually and painful during menstruation, if your uterus seems to be your enemy, you'll be surprised by this wonderful, beautiful journey into your womb. If you are already comfortable with your womb and bleeding time, this journey will increase your connection.

Relax. Envision or imagine yourself becoming smaller and smaller. See yourself lying on the bed or the floor with slightly-parted legs.

Once you're small enough, gently climb between the lips of your vagina. Look around. Carefully touch the skin. Inhale and smell.

Now go slowly down the dark red, pink, brown corridor that leads to the womb. Feel your way forward. Little trickles of blood run under your feet, through the corridor, outwards. Enter the uterus through your cervix.

At first, it's tight, then there's more room and it's more comfortable. You can even stand up. Note the texture, color and shape of the walls of your womb. Feel the blood that rains from the ceiling and runs down the walls.

Hum or speak and listen to the echo. Lay yourself down on the soft, velvety floor of your uterus and listen to your body's sounds: the beating of your heart, the songs of the intestinal tract, the whoosh of your breath. Look and feel carefully. Where is your uterus cramped? Where is it soft and loose? [What does your womb tell you? What does it want or need?]

When you've been in your womb long enough, let yourself be carried out with the menstrual blood. Once out, imagine you're growing, becoming bigger, and finally you are once again full size. Stretch slowly as before, and make a record of your experiences.

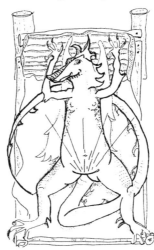

Dragontime Dances

I first connected to menstrual (trance) dancing through the dance of the Menaden (see my book, *Mond, Tanz, Magie*) and through bacchanals (named after Bacchus, the god of wine). At ancient bacchanals participants danced excitedly until they fell down, exhausted, tension released, and minds open to insights and visions. This type of dance goes much further back in myth then Bacchus does though; perhaps all the way back to ancient menstrual rituals. The Spring Solstice 1981 issue of "Womanspirit" describes an ancient spring ritual that suggests these roots: Greek women used to celebrate the menstruating goddess and the newly awakened fertility of the earth (and women) by dancing during *Anthesters*.

These ancient menstrual dances have become known by many names: shamanic dances, initiation dances, the tarantella of Italy. It's good to dance during menstruation. Our ancestresses knew that the uterus relaxes when other muscles work and that menstrual pain and tension are eased quickly by movement and dance.

Stamping

Stamping on the ground is the basic step for menstrual dances. Stamp in a regular easy rhythm, from one foot to the other. You can do it alone, but it's especially wonderful to do with a group of women. Don't speed up, though you may get louder and louder.

Try stamping with bells on one ankle. Try it moving sideways.
In addition to simple stamping, add voice: stamp left, stamp right,
then say "Wha" or "Whoo." Let it come from the belly and be
strengthened by the stamping. Let it be a fully satisfying sound. Let a
threefold beat develop: Left, right, "Wha." Left, right, "Wha!"

Dragon Dance

Form a circle of women. [Focus together on a mutual intention or
on each woman's personal needs.] Begin stamping: left, right, left, right.
Then develop a three-fold beat: left, right, "Wha," left, right, "Wha."
Keep to this rhythm, on and on, on and on. When it has worked its
way into you strongly and deeply, stamp slowly toward the middle until
you're standing very close to each other. Continue stamping with the
same rhythm, but do it very close: left, and right, and "Wha!" from
the belly with all your might. Take some time to concentrate the energy
in the middle. At a signal [when the cone of power is raised and released],
everyone turns around to face out of the circle and stamps out left,
right, "Wha." Then turning left, all stamp three times around the circle.
The rhythm stays the same all the way through this dance, but as it
ends (the last time around the circle), the sounds grow quieter and the
movements softer, until all stand still.

Humming Circle

All women lie in a circle. Each one lies with her head between the
legs of the next with another woman's head in her lap, one woman
after another. When the circle is closed, everyone starts to hum deeply,
a humming circle from belly to head, head to belly develops. (Thank
you, Christa-Marie!)

Cradle

A woman with abdominal pain or one who simply wants to relax,
can be rocked from side to side by two other women. Stand opposite
one another, rocking her back and forth. She must always keep both
feet firmly on the floor, but otherwise can relax and give her whole
body over to the two women.

Sister Support

Divide into groups of two. Women lean softly against each other,
back to back, keeping spines straight. Rub back and bottom, neck and

head; rub softly on each other. Be so relaxed that if you weren't leaning against each other, your head and neck would loll around on each other's shoulder. Enjoy it for a long time.

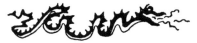

Dragontime Dance Ritual

The women meet on a wonderfully hot night out in the open country. The women meet on cold night in a big private room in the city which can stand up to some active dancing! Each woman brings her menstrual amulet or her power necklace or her rag dress, something which represents and reminds her of the power of her menstruation.

The women who dance in this ritual don't need to be menstruating. They are celebrating their dragon power. [Women who no longer bleed and women without their uterus dance and celebrate, too.]

In the middle of the circle an altar is built. Feathers, stones, woven baskets, flowers, buds, fruit, seeds, pictures, dragon dolls, clay figures, bloody rags, and the personal menstrual power objects brought by each woman are arranged there. Each woman has painted and ornamented herself. On a large table women place what they've brought to eat and drink.

When all the preparations are finished, the food laid out nicely, and the altar glowing with candles, the painted and ornamented women form a circle. All join hands. Each woman in turn offers a word describing the energy she brings in, her feelings, her important thoughts.

Four women have planned in advance to evoke the directions of the compass. One woman turns towards the east and calls out: "I call you, energy of the east, clear air, wind, intuition, guardian of thoughts." [Or, of course, an invocation of her own, ending with "Be here now."]

One woman turns to the south and calls: "I call you, woman of the south, heat, fire, brewing and boiling, guardian of the cauldron." ["Be here now."]

One woman turns to the west and calls out: "I call you, beings of the west, soft energy, water, the depths of the ocean, guardian of the bitter waters and the sweet springs, and of blood." ["Be here now."]

The last woman turns to the north: "I call you, spirits of the north, darkness of the night, solidity of the earth, warm shelter guardian of caves and mountains." ["Be here now."]

Then, all together the women call in the four elemental sisters (air, fire, water, earth) with screams, chirps and twitters, growls and snarls, barks and purrs, howls, hisses and hums.

The sounds give way to silence. Everyone waits.

One woman moves. She stamps: left, right, left, right. The rest of the circle joins and the rhythm is intensified with voices and hands. One or more women take up drums and drum the peaceful, even, dependable rhythm of blood: left, right, left, right. Heartbeat. Womb-beat. [Add a chant or a wordless "hummmm. . . ."]

When the rhythm is established, the circle moves slowly left. From this point on, any woman who wants can move inside the circle dance however she wants. She may dance to the four elements, the altar, the drummers, the other women, herself, to menstrual mysteries, to anything.

The dance comes to an end as women get tired. The circling to the left stops, the drumbeat ceases. Women stamp quietly together: left, right, and stop. [If you're at all dizzy touch your hands and forehead to the earth.]

Finish with a feast. [Share stories of your dragontime while you eat.]

The celebration draws to an end, night comes, night goes, and the women change slowly, almost imperceptibly, but ceaselessly.

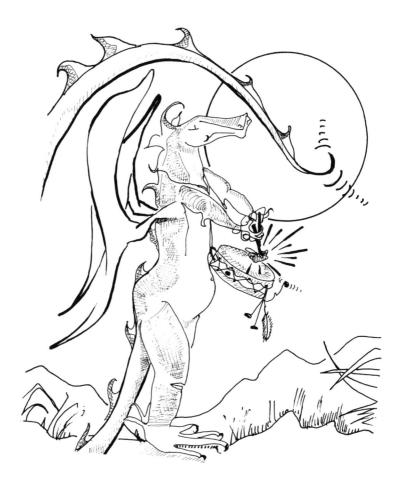

Dragontime Exercises

[These exercises are part of dragontime mysteries. They're effective and fun, alone or in a small group. And—to show you just how they're done—we're proud to introduce Mau Blossom's friend, Zabu.]

Embrace the Moon, as well as the Accordion Squeeze are good to the belly, helping it and the back to get lots of oxygen.

Embrace the Moon

Stand with legs spread hip width. Bend softly at the knees and pull in your pelvis, so that your back is straight. The outer leg muscles are tensed while the muscles of the inner leg and the vagina are relaxed.

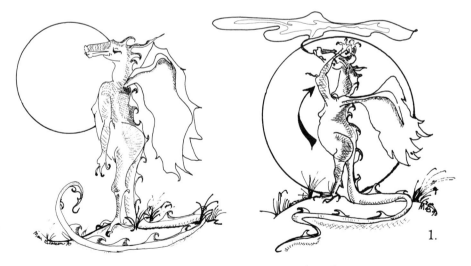

1. Breathe in, lift both arms in front of you with palms down, up over your head until palms face front.

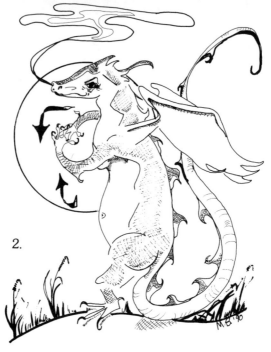

2. Breathe out, slowly dropping the arms forward to form a circle in front of you, as though the moon was there in front of your belly and you could embrace it.

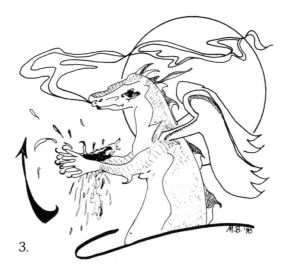

3. Then turn your palms up and as you breathe in, imagine you're scooping up water in front of your body, over your shoulders, and up to your head.

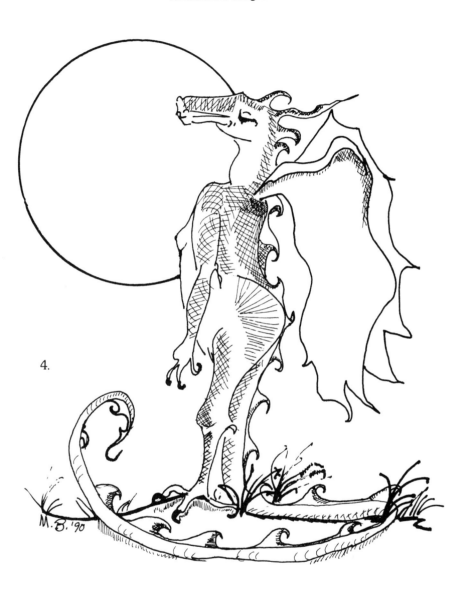

4.

M.B. '90

4. As you breathe out again, let your hands and arms spread out to the sides and sink, palms up. Imagine water flowing out in a fountain around you as the arms stretch out to the sides and down.

In brief: Breathe in, lift arms up, high but loose. Breathe out, embrace the moon. Breathe in, scoop up water. Breathe out, let the water flow out around you.

Accordion Squeeze

An advanced variation of: Inhale, arms high. Exhale, all fall down. [In its most basic form, you may have done this exercise: inhale, raise your arms; exhale, hands to toes.] Stand with legs hip width, feet firm, spine and head aligned.

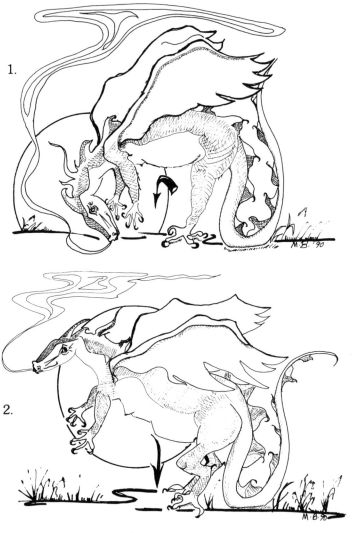

1. Breathe in, arms down, bend upper body slowly at the hips.
2. Breathe out, let the whole body sink into a squat, as far down as you can go and still keep your feet flat on the floor (not on tip toe).

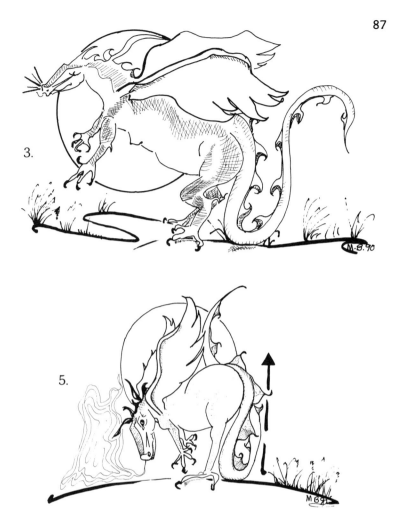

3.

5.

3. When all the air is squeezed out of your body push the rest out through your nose with a short blow. (Exhaling is more important than inhaling. Once there's no air left in the body, it spontaneously takes in a breath on its own.)

4. As you inhale, draw your breath into your back, and stretch your head and spine up, keeping the butt down.

5. Exhale, straighten the legs and push your butt up. Now you're standing with legs straight, upper body bent over the floor.

6. Inhale and straighten up.

In brief: Inhale, bend forward with your upper body and arms. Breathe out slowly, pull your whole body down like an accordion onto your calves, with your feet flat on the ground. Squeeze the air out. Breathe in, straighten up from the hips. Breathe out, push up with the legs, nose down. Breathe in: slowly straighten upper body.

Belly Breath

Here's a yoga exercise for relieving back pain during your period. It is a powerful strengthener for the belly. (Backaches are often caused by weak belly muscles: the back compensates for the belly, and gets overstrained.)

This breathing exercise can also be done before a ritual. Oxygen fuels the magical fires.

Stand with your knees loose and legs spread out at about hip-breadth.

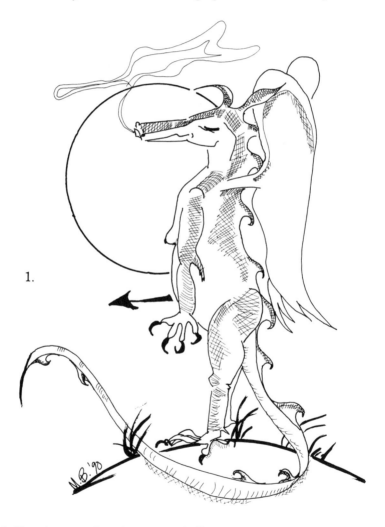

1. Breathe in and push out your belly.

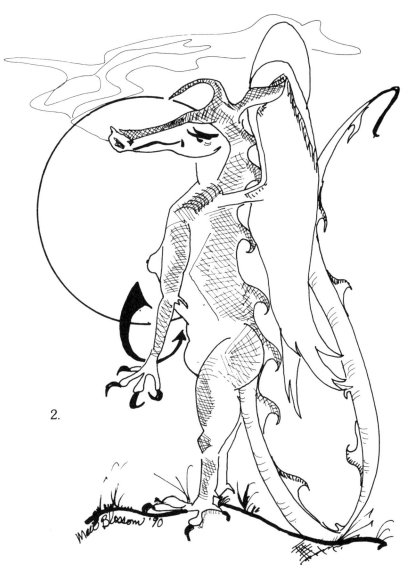

2.

2. Breathe out and pull your belly in towards your back bone.
3. When there's no air left, without breathing, pull your belly up under your ribs to form a kind of vacuum. Hold [a few seconds at first, gradually increasing to no more than 6 seconds. For extra energy, clench the anal and vaginal muscles while holding the breath out. Relax them before inhaling.]

Belly Dances

Note that in all these exercises the feet should be firmly on the ground. Contact with the earth gives strength and is very important for the uterus and belly.

Do these as loosely as you can. Don't strain. Relax. Enjoy. Belly pain is diminished by soft and joyful movements. Keep some tension on the outer side of the leg, if you wish, as this can help to relax the inner leg and vaginal muscles.

• Belly circles: Stand with your legs about three feet/one meter apart, feet flat on the ground. Imagine that you're standing in a gigantic bowl. Your belly, hips and butt make a circle by sliding around the inside of the bowl. Trace big sweeping circles with the belly. Bend lightly at the knees so the hips can move more easily. Circle left. Circle right.

• Figure Eights: Push one hip forward, then out to the side, then back, then forward again. Then push the other hip forward, to the side, backward then forward again. Each half of the figure eight begins forward, goes to the side and back, then returns to the normal position of the body. If this is too complicated for you, then just rock your hips to the right and left.

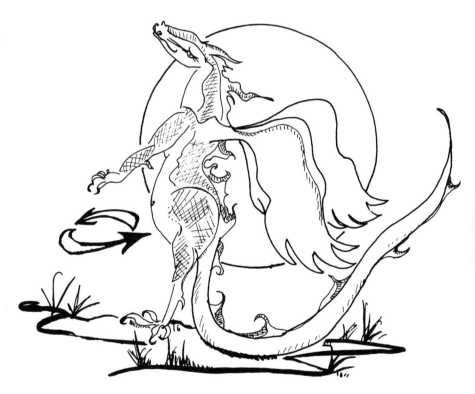

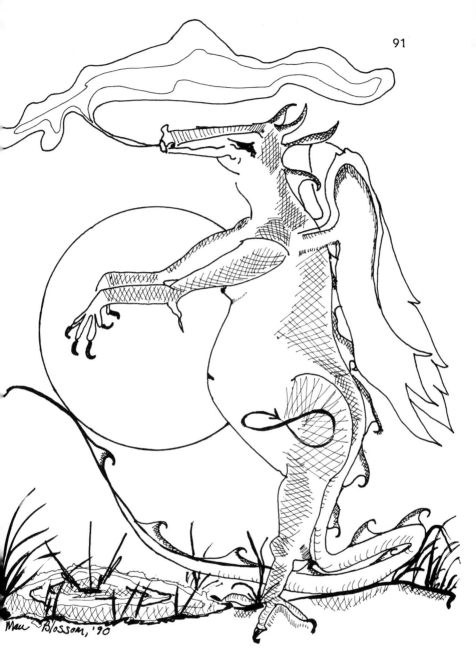

• Pelvic Rocks: Tip your pelvis back and forth while standing in the usual position. Really push your butt out toward the back. While you're doing it, let go of the thought that it's obscene. The more pronounced and sensual the movement, the better it is for your abdomen.

As these movements become easier for you, start doing them while walking forward. That can result in an endless variety of beautiful dances!

Belly Chakra Exercise

Stand on one side of a room. [Attach an imaginary filament from the wall to your belly button.] Draw both arms up in front of your body, threateningly, as though ready to strike or defend. Concentrate on your belly button. Then, left, right, "Wha!," stamp across the room. Strike the arms and hands forward with conscious decisive movements. Let out any sound that comes up in you. Breathe from your belly.

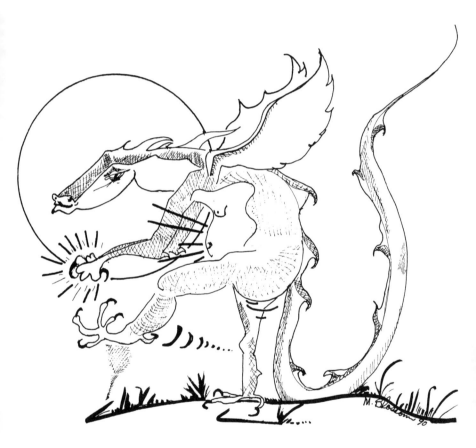

Windmill and Soft Shoulders help relieve tension carried by the shoulders. A looser neck and shoulders means less menstrual cramping.

Windmill

Stand with legs spread about hip width, bending softly at the knees.
1. Breathe in, tip your pelvis forward. Swing your right arm towards the back, up, and over, then down to the front. Simultaneously, swing the left arm in the opposite direction: to the front, up, and over, then down to the back.
2. Breathe out, let the pelvis relax.
3. Repeat the whole exercise, arms going in opposite directions.

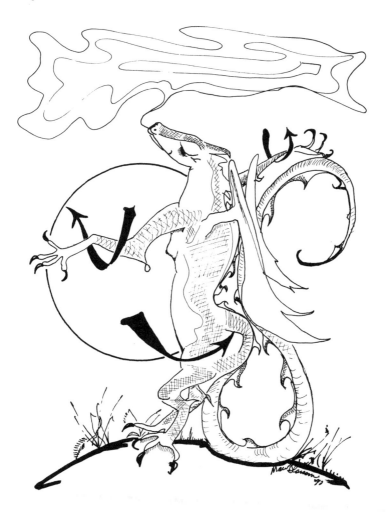

Soft Shoulders

1. Stand firmly, feet fully in touch with the ground, arms loose.
2. Breathe in, pull the shoulders up to the ears, then the left shoulder goes forward, the right shoulder goes back; both drop down, towards the armpit, then left moves back, right moves front.
3. Inhale, shoulders are up, continue.

Perhaps it sounds complicated but the idea of a staff running across and through both shoulders around which they circle makes it easier. After a while, reverse direction.

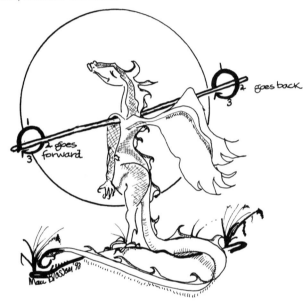

Toad

Crouch down on the floor like a toad, breasts pressed against your thighs, feet flat on the floor. (Do Accordion Squeeze first to loosen thighs.) Slowly, like a toad, stretch the body up and then down again onto the thighs. This relieves abdominal cramps and draws a lot of oxygen into the belly. Try it quickly too, like a frog.

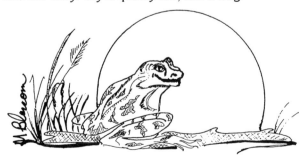

Vaginal Breath

If you've no energy for exercise, lie down comfortably in bed. Make it cozy and pleasant for yourself. Breathe and relax. Open your legs and imagine you're breathing through your vagina, your belly, your womb.

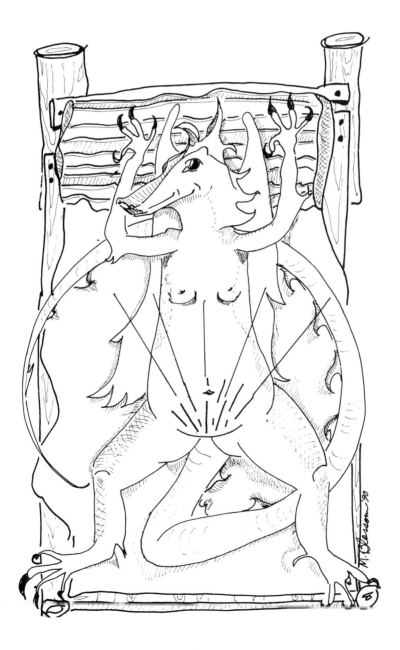

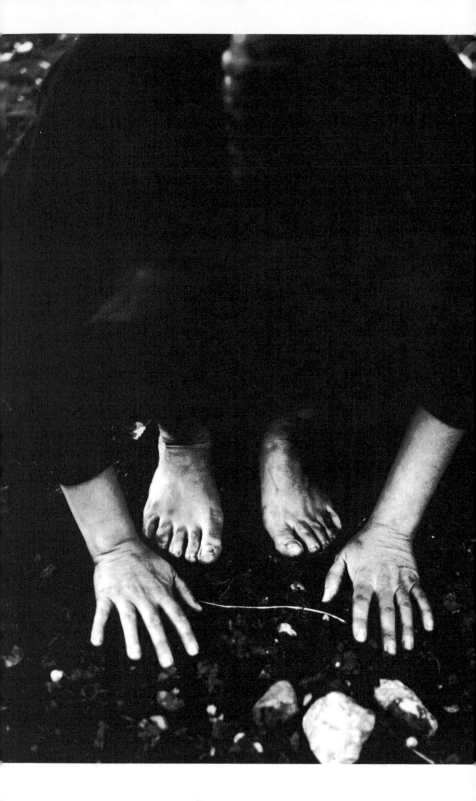

Dragontime Rituals

The trinity of maiden (menarche), mother (menstruation), and crone (menopause) is the great life cycle of women, the triad of menstruation, and the ancient triple moon goddesses: Persephone, Demeter, and Hecate. [The spiraling of this trinity is enhanced by—and enhances—all rituals.]

The Dragon Maiden

The young woman before menstruating is the maiden. Her color is white. Her home is in the air or the sky. She can fly. The dragon maiden, not yet initiated into womanly responsibilities, is still wild and free, like Artemis. Still a child, she is yet a woman.

In fairy tales, her story goes like this:

The oddest thing about the maiden is that she doesn't just pack her bags and leave the country. After all, she's to be sacrificed to the dragon who's already polished off all the other maidens of the land.

But the dragon maiden doesn't leave. Instead she's determined not to be made the exception. The king wants her spared and the prince, Sir Highness himself, courageously offers to challenge the monster, but the princess doesn't want their help and doesn't even seem to be terribly frightened. How can that be possible?

Could she suspect that her initiation into womanhood will take place on this exciting day? That entering the cave of the dragon will change her?

As we immerse ourselves in the dragon tales in which maidens are sacrificed it becomes clear that they are actually describing initation rites. In African girls' puberty rites, the young women are grabbed by a woman in a demon mask, and they have to resist her.

What sort of special thing awaits our maiden? Is it dragon blood? Is it a special little universe, an ecosystem in and of itself? Beyond the balance of men having a penis, and women having a clitoris, women have a special private world of bleeding. Women can build up and let go, give life and bring death, all in one monthly cycle.

The dragon maiden is the child-woman who is learning, becoming ready to be introduced to a new reality, a mythical world [and the opening of special powers of vision, healing, wisdom, and foreknowledge]. Western, white-identified cultures have moved completely away from this idea. When young, dominant culture women bleed for the first time, it's either noted from a distance, or commented on negatively: "So you've got it now, too. You poor thing. Oh, well, you can't escape it."

In modern patriarchal cultures, a young woman's first menstruation makes her accessible and endangered. Now she's considered "sexually mature," and from this point on she has to "watch out" not to attract men, or "get herself" pregnant. Men claim this as the specific point in time at which a woman's sexuality and eroticism begin, as if dragon maidens previously had no sexuality and now need men to complete them sexually.

The first bleeding for a modern young woman is the beginning of being told (and eventually feeling) that a woman is "only half a person." Instead of initiation, there's struggle. From now on you must strive to be a pair, to feel yourself to be part of a pair, even if the other part is nowhere in sight. Becoming a woman changes into becoming a wife. Not experiencing your own body, but giving it to your husband and children.

What was your initiation?

The dragon maiden who is secure in her power experiences her first blood with a mixture of sadness as childhood passes, and joy mingled with fear as she's accepted into the women's circle. She grows, opens the thirteenth door, steps over the threshold, and finds her fingers bloody. She is celebrated.

Dragon maidens of today are beginning to want wonderful celebrations, too. Will we create our own women's rituals again? Will we supplant the endless communions and confirmations? Will we become our own dragon selves again?

A Ritual Celebration for the Dragon Maiden

Celebrate sometime during the first year of a young woman's bleeding with a wonderful white party.

The maiden wears a white dress. At the celebration, everyone adds red or rose-red trim: flowers, buds, lace, ribbon. Let it be fantastic and beautiful. Let it evoke the part of every woman that wants to be a princess. Now's the time when the princess takes power!

For the meal have only white and pink foods, such as strawberries and cream, turkey and cranberries, raspberries and yogurt.

To symbolize the maiden's new status as a dragon who bleeds, the dragon mothers and maidens make a birth canal and carry her through it to a new birth. Have two women stand facing each other, then another pair, and another stand by them, until as long a line as possible is formed. The maiden to be initiated is lifted into the arms of the first pair of women and—feet first—rocked down the entire line. At the end she's picked up and kissed by her mother or a crone (woman who no longer bleeds).

The birth canal can be created in two other ways. Either: all the women stand one behind the other with their legs spread wide and the dragon maiden crawls through and emerges as a dragon who bleeds. Or: the women stand across from each other as before, only closer, belly to belly. The dragon maiden must wind her way between the bellies (surely a soft, loving journey). I think the most pleasant birth is to be rocked through.

Then let there be drumming, dancing, feasting and celebrating.

The Dragon Mother

The woman who bleeds, the fertile woman in the fullness of her life is the mother. Her color is red. Her realm is the abundant earth. She's the dragon mother, fruitful and frightful at the same time, in the bloom of her life. (In the middle ages menstruation was also called the bloom, and women who were depicted in a flower garden, symbolically represent the bleeding fruitful woman.)

The dragon mother is the woman at the peak of her fertility, a fertility not limited to bearing children. How might we imagine fertility in other ways? Creative energy, perhaps? I think of women engaged in weaving, building, cooking, and celebrating. I think of times when it was a primary task to encourage nature's fertility so she would provide enough for nourishment and the necessities of life. Yes, creativity and fertility are the same. (Until I think of today's skyscrapers or acrylic sweaters or canned food then creativity seems far from fertility.)

I know my fertility as a joyful life force, as a desire to make things happen, as my ability to make visible my dreams and visions. But I don't feel much support or space or time for that. It's complicated and difficult for me to live out the life of dragon mother.

The dragon mother is the menstruating, mature woman. She spits fire, a symbol for blood. In a less metaphorical sense, she's the raging, aggressive, charged-up woman.

She lives in a cave, by herself, at one with herself, woven into her own time. Her cave is warm, dark, protected, unapproachable. She has sulphur on her skin, a dangerous yellow gaze in her eyes, and an impatient twitch when disturbed.

During menstruation, many women withdraw into memories, pulling back into their caves. How pleasant to draw back, fleeing to the end of time and over the edge of the world, out to the island of memory.

Imagine then some little brat, spoiling for a dragon fight, wanting very much to stick his sword in somewhere to get at blood! That makes the dragon mother's fire burn out of control, perhaps hurting others in the vicinity. The family pulls back. Fiery blazes of rage, depression, despair, and pain flare up.

Approach dragon mothers with special care. They live apart from normal social niceties. Dragontime, menstruation, is the last remnant of undomesticated woman.

When I hurt in some way or another during menstruation I'm happy that I have a physical, palpable link to the old powers, the blood mysteries, menstrual magic. More important to me now than anything else is learning to access these powers, to understand these realities.

Solitary Dragontime Ritual

Use your menstrual blood to add power to ritual. Go to a beautiful spot in nature, preferably protected and remote so you won't be disturbed. Take with you four objects to represent the four directions or elements. I lay out: something for the air in the east [feathers, incense, flute], something for the fire in the south [cauldron, corn, drum], something for the earth in the west [crystal, tobacco, rattle], something for water in the north [cup, juice, harp].

Circle once [or more] around the ritual place you've set up. [Circle clockwise (sunwards), to gather energy for your circle. Circle counterclockwise (widdershins), to release energy from your circle. Note also, I put water in the west, earth in the north. Others do it other ways. In New Zealand/Australia, north is usually fire. What feels right to you? Do it!]

Envision your intention. Call to your circle the energies, archetypes, animal allies, goddesses, and powers that can help you. Sing, dance, visualize, pray. In the middle of your circle make a fire. A little one of fragrant herbs or twigs in a cauldron will do if conditions prohibit something larger. Once the fire's burning put your menstrual blood (or a piece of paper with your blood on it) into the fire. Concentrate on [and open up to] the desired change.

Honor your menstrual blood and your intention as powerful forces. Rule out doubt and resignation. Spread clarity within yourself. Wish that all may benefit.

When the fire's burned down, thank your helpers, pick up any objects you don't want to leave, release the circle, and leave. (Is the fire really out?)

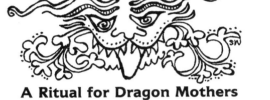

A Ritual for Dragon Mothers

Invite your women friends for a dragon party. Decorate with red and some occasional sulfur yellow: red paintings, red candles, red food. Everyone wears raggedy red clothes. An ancient custom in the Alps, and in several African cultures, is wearing "the rag skirt," "the fool's skirt," "the coat of many colors," which symbolizes all energies gathered together. [Symbolic of being on the "rag"?]

Create a sacred circle and chant or drum to stir your energy. Then women jump into the circle, trilling, twittering, whistling, and screeching. Some have little bells on their legs and on their clothes. For awhile, everyone jumps and runs around in the circle, screaming, letting out deep, grunting sounds, hissing, roaring, interspersed with other simple sounds like "ha" and "ho." Then one after the other jumps into a permanent place in the circle. Everyone joins hands.

One begins, saying her name (it might be one she wishes she had). Now everyone sings, screams, whispers, and says this name. So it goes, around the circle, until everyone has been named.

Then the women circle tightly, pressed up close, each behind the next. Every butt melts into the belly of the woman behind it. Everyone moves in until the circle is closed. In the style of the ancient dance, which has been handed down to us from as long ago as the wall paintings of the Tassili mountains in Algeria, 4000 years before our record of time, every woman bends far forward, loose in the knees, to make soft swings with every step, back and forth, hips all the way to the right, all the way to the left, in synchrony with the other women. Rock as a single being, feel the body of the women in front and behind you, melt together, rock each other, enjoy.

If you're outside, build a fire. You can jump over it. You can nourish it by giving it something—a scream or sentence (it's nice if it rhymes), a chant, a written phrase on a bit of paper or birch bark. You can dance around it. With a group of women, I once danced such a fire dance that became ever more joyous and wild. So wild, we wanted to walk through the fire. It was a wonderful experience: we stepped, excited and joyful, into the fire, and at the end danced it out.

[Spend some time sharing dragontime stories. Then home to your dreams.]

The Dragon Crone

The old woman, the woman who no longer bleeds, is the crone. She is the goddess of the crossroads, the one who has experienced all three phases of a woman's life, who knows much, and who is acquainted with many things. Her color is black. (In Italy and Greece all old women wear black.)

Her domain is the ocean, the watery deeps. She's the dragon crone who's given birth to, lived as, and left behind the dragon maiden and the dragon mother. The dragon crone is the guardian of wisdom. She keeps watch over secrets. On the search for treasure or the quest for the beloved, every road leads to her. She can hinder you, block your way, kill you, or allow you to pass.

Stories and tales from around the world tell us that the path to knowledge leads through the old woman, the old witch, the devil's grandmother, the old woods-woman, the dragon crone. She seems so fragile, but, when it matters, is astonishingly agile. The crone is unpredictable, bad-tempered, and foolish. No one takes her seriously and then suddenly she shows her power. The heroes of fairy tales have to work things out with the dragon crone before they can even think about the maiden.

The old crone grandmother knows the secrets of time, space, and other worlds. The dragon crone knows where the beloved of the hero is hidden. The beloved is often a maiden who's come to apprentice with the crone. She knows where the treasure lies. The path to her lair takes "maybe days, maybe years, who knows."

The crone usually lives in a little house in the woods, and speaks with the moon or the wind. She can call them, just like friends, or even whistle them up if she has the need. In one fairy tale, in fact, we find her living in a little cottage which turns with the wind on a weather vane.

When meeting the fairy tale hero, she almost always comments that she hasn't smelled Christian flesh for a long time, for she embodies the time before patriarchal religions and the domestication of women.

In one fairy tale, a princess is exiled when she tells her father, the king, that she loves him as much as salt. The crone becomes her guardian. This crone makes the prince (who wishes to free the princess) work for her. First she asks him to carry her. She becomes so heavy he thinks he'll collapse under her weight. But at last he accomplishes everything to her satisfaction and she brings him and the princess together.

The dragon crone has the power to protect maiden and mother dragons. She shares her experience and wisdom. Who can tell young women what awaits them if not the crone? Who knows thoroughly the weaknesses and lies of the system? The crone! And who's no longer afraid to speak out? The crone!

Why has the crone been cast as a monster, evil and ugly? Why are old women so frequently treated badly in myths and fairy tales? Because it is her power that the patriarchs fear above all others. The crone doesn't feel the need to change herself anymore to "pass," no longer feels compelled to please. She pleases herself, acting from her own wisdom, her own experience.

The dragon crone is the sole owner of her wise blood. Freed from the awesome responsibility of nourishing another life within herself, she nourishes where she pleases and what she pleases.

Feast for the Ancestresses

Meet for a dinner party or picnic. Every woman brings an ancestress or goddess with her. When the table is being set, every woman has a place for herself and a place for the ancient one she's invited.

Sit in a circle. One by one, describe who you have brought and why. Then share the food. Ideally, the plates for the ancestresses are allowed to stay full. (Although, on occasions of great hunger, I've been known to eat for my ancestress too, and it's done me good.)

I've found that the ancestresses prefer grains, honey, milk, blood, and fruit. This is also the wisdom that's been passed down through the ages about them.

You can go alone and feast the ancestresses in the woods. You'll soon receive visits from wild animals, especially if there's salad (without dressing, of course) and seeds laying around.

In Africa, ancestress spirits are associated with millet and with saliva. If you gather herbs, cut wood, or dig roots, remember the ancient ones by spitting or leaving millet seeds.

A Ritual for Dragon Crones

Who wants to be fruitful forever? The bleeding time stops, reminding every woman of something many would like to deny: we are all mortal. Time passes, and the snake sheds her skin. That time is coming—are we ready? Have we learned what we came to learn, have we done what we came to do? Ursula LeGuin says menopause is our best and only chance to become a wise old woman.

At this time, a connection to other self-loving women is especially important. Let the end of menstruation be celebrated together.

Let dragon mothers, dragon maidens, and dragon crones meet for a party to celebrate wisdom gained and destiny satisfied. The dragon crones dress in black, accented with the colors of the sea and the moon. The dragon maidens dress in white clothes trimmed with red or pink. The dragon mothers dress in red and yellow rags or feathered clothes. All the women bring a favorite cup (or bowl) for holding a small amount of water.

Work together to prepare a great feast which features plants from the nightshade family: tomatoes, potatoes, eggplant, peppers of all colors.

In the center of the area of celebration set a cauldron (or large pot) filled with water. Each woman sets her cup next to the cauldron.

All the women join in a circle around the cauldron and begin to stamp out a beat: even, strong, restful.

When the energy has focused in the circle, all the women stamp into the middle of the circle, tight around the cauldron. Then the dragon crones pick up their cups, and dip water from the cauldron and sip, saying, "I accept the wisdom of ages past." The dragon maidens and mothers then pick up their cups, dip and drink, saying also, "I accept the wisdom of ages past."

Then the dragon mothers and maidens set their cup back down by the cauldron and move back. The crones stay close to the cauldron. One by one each crone says or sings the important wisdom she has learned in her life, the most satisfying accomplishments. As each thing is named, the crone pours a little water from her cup back into the cauldron, adding to the wisdom of the ages. Time passes. The wisdom and deeds of the crones weave a powerful web of strength in the room.

When all the crones are done talking of their past, they begin to name the wisdom they still need or things they still want to do to complete their destiny. As each one names something, another crone dips water from the cauldron and gives it to her to sip, or pours a little over her head, saying as she does, "Take from the goddess's wise cauldron the patience you seek" (or the strength to accomplish something, or whatever). "Shed the skin that has become too tight for you and be born anew."

When the crones are done, the maidens and mothers may ask for what they need to accomplish their destiny. A crone gives water to sip or pours a little over the head, repeating: "Take (whatever she needs) from the goddess's cauldron. Shed the skin that has become too tight for you and be born anew."

When the seeking is completed, the dragon crones join hands, forming an inner circle around the cauldron. The dragon maidens and mothers join hands forming an outer circle. At first the crones alone circle the cauldron, moving left. Then the maidens and mothers in the outer ring begin to stamp around the circle to the right, keeping an even steady rhythm. Time passes. The dragon crones move around the cauldron to the left. The dragon mothers to the right, stamping. The women in both circles begin to make noises: hisses, hoots, howls, whatever comes up. Then all the crones stand still, while the maidens and mothers continue to circle, stamping.

At a signal, all become quiet. The dragon maidens and mothers in the outer circle raise up their joined hands and stamp into the middle of the circle until they reach the dragon crones. The crones slip under the raised hands and join hands in a large circle on the outside. Raising hands, they move in again and make one circle with the mothers and maidens.

Holding hands they circle the cauldron a few times, then break the circle by covering their solar plexus with their hands. Afterwards the women may want to go to the cauldron to dip out more wisdom to drink or to take home and set on their altar.

Use the water that's left during the rest of your celebration: to make a soup for all to eat, or, in the summer, to cool off, or . . . . When done, pour what's left back into the earth.

Another beautiful ritual is one I found in *Womanspirit*, 1982 Fall Equinox issue, by Portia Cornell of Canton, Connecticut.

> The Ceremony attracted twenty women. We gathered in a room with a vaginal fire on the hearth at the opening of the circle. When we all gathered we spoke of the specialness of this occasion. We had time for meditation. Then we wove a strand of yarn binding us together: red for menstruation, black for death, and golden for wisdom. We said: "This is the blood that binds all women together."
>
> We passed the conch shell and each woman spoke her mind. The menopausal women (there were six) sat in the center of the circle with hemlock wreaths on their heads. They looked both wonderful and glowing and slightly comical with the branches jutting out every which way. We all cackled and then gave them a rousing applause. They beamed. They began to speak of the wisdom they knew. I felt like a little girl . . . listening . . . as the elder women of the tribe passed on their wisdom.
>
> We were healing ourselves of our fears and loneliness through sharing combined with ritual. Then we each tossed a seed, nut or egg into the fire and told what we were letting go of. We then did a birth line such as is traditional on candlemas. . . . Some of the babies bucked their way through. Some screamed their way

through. The mothers patted their buttocks. "It's a girl!" we kept yelling as each one emerged . . . then the African drum music began and we feasted and danced. I felt that the Ceremony, preceded by all the sharing we had done in the group, was, as in the early religious ceremonies, truly transformative . . . an electrifying experience.

Another good custom is for the wise crones, the women on the other side of menstruation, to become godmothers to young women and have festivals where they pass along to this woman everything that's important to them. In this way, when it's time, power objects can be handed on and the net between women can become denser and more capable of supporting us.

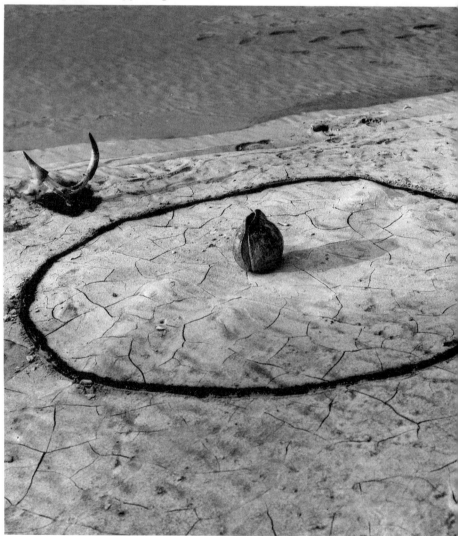

DRAGONTIME
Future Visions

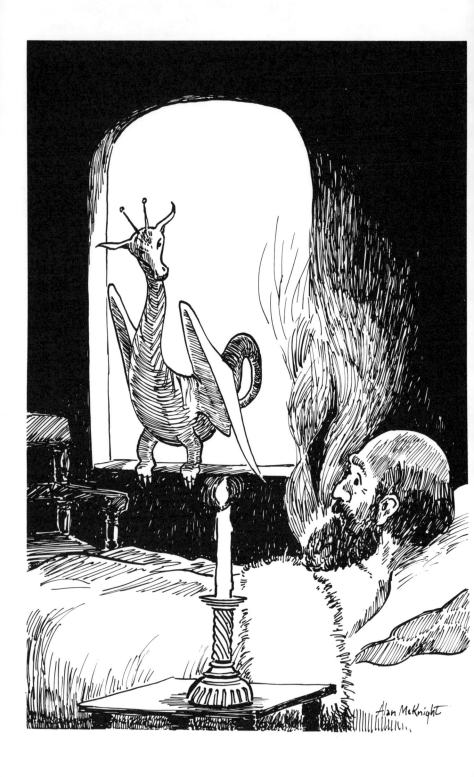

Future Visions: Reweaving the Magic and Mystery

"The Maidens and the Dragons"

When fall came, the king looked out the window full of worry. At the new moon the maiden sacrifice would come due, and there were no young girls left in the land besides his own daughter. The sacrifice of maidens was a dark chapter of his rule. Barely had he conquered the land, taken the queen to be his wife, and sent his troops out across the land, than this old woman had come to speak with him. He wanted to send her away, but suddenly she stood in the middle of the throne room. "Behead her," he yelled, enraged. But his men, seized by a strangely petrifying horror, were unable to move.

"I am the grandmother of the dragon and ancestress of the queen whom you killed," said the crone. He tried to brush aside the thought of his lovely wife, who had jumped from the tower, to escape belonging to him. "If you do not bring an innocent maiden every year after the harvest to the dragon cave at Dragonstone, then dragons will come and destroy your land with fire."

With that she was gone.

Of course, he put no stock in the confusing speech of this old enchantress. He didn't even consider fulfilling the requirement. Not because he felt any compassion for the girls, but because he, the king, would not let himself be coerced by an old woman. He proclaimed a celebration. There was drinking and singing and people fell under the old oak table. Fall came. No girl was brought to the dragon cave.

But once the leaves had fallen and the night of the full moon arrived, suddenly, at midnight, a little dragon sat on the king's window sill.

"Where is the maiden?" rasped the dragon, and with every word a blast of fire issued forth, ate its way across the room, through the furs on the king, to the hairs of his beard.

He sprang wide awake. The dragon sailed away from the window and was quickly lost to sight in the distance. The room of the king looked like the aftermath of a battle. He tore at what was left of his hair, forced to realize that there *were* such things as dragons and that he and all his soldiers were powerless against them. He had it proclaimed across the land that a maiden should be brought to him without delay. As none came voluntarily, he sent out his soldiers. They grabbed a maiden and, as hard as she struggled and cried, it was of no help to her. She had to go to the dragon cave.

A long mourning procession accompanied her: her crying parents, her friends, the members of the king's court, and, at the end, the people.

At the entrance of the cave stood the grandmother and she took the girl into her possession. Then the two of them disappeared into the cave and were never seen again.

Year after year it proceeded so. When the leaves had fallen, and the moon was full, a maiden was taken to the dragon's cave. Fathers fell into panic, hid their daughters or sent them out of the country. Curiously enough, the girls were growing less and less afraid. It was told of the smith's daughter that on the night before she'd been taken to the cave, she dreamed of all the maidens of the land awaiting her at Dragonstone and having a great party to celebrate the occasion of her arrival. At the party the dragon's grandmother, in reality the old queen, gave out star-shaped flowers to all.

"Fate is kind to her," the people whispered. "She's no longer right in her head."

While the king sat at the window, growling, the princess sat in her room and bedecked herself. She put on her most beautiful dress. That afternoon she'd woven a wreath of field flowers, which she now set upon her black hair. "Be patient, my friends. I'm now coming to join you. My father tried to smuggle me out of the country, but I set up such a fuss that he soon gave up his plan."

Suddenly someone knocked on the door. A young man stood outside. He was excited. "Princess, I'll save you. I'll kill the dragon and take you as my bride," he announced, and pulled his sword out of its scabbard and laid it at her feet.

She shoved the sword a little to the side with her toe. "We'll see," she said. "You can come with me to the dragon's cave. The rest will become clear in time."

The prince bowed down deeply in front of her and disappeared.

Soon it was time to go. A servant, however, had been eavesdropping at the princess' door and knew of the prince's plan. He himself was in love with the princess, so he decided to let the prince fight the dragon but go himself to the king to receive the reward when the dragon was dead. He stealthily followed the mourning procession, led by the princess and her lady's-maid, followed by the king in war-like garb and by soldiers in four columns, who sang blood-chilling songs. At the back, as always, came the people, who were amazed at the beauty and liveliness of the princess.

When they all arrived at the dragon's cave (which shimmered silver in the light of the full moon) a tearful farewell was taken. The minstrels and jugglers composed songs about the event and departed immediately to spread the news that the princess now resided with the dragons. Suddenly, the dragon grandmother stood in the middle of the cave, dressed in a dark cloak, and stretched her arms out to the princess. Lamenting and screaming loudly, the whole crowd departed.

Not so the brave prince . . . nor the servant, who had hidden himself behind a bush. The prince drew out his sword and yelled, "Show yourself, you cowardly dragon and I'll vanquish you!"

Hardly had he spoken the words when a dragon came crawling out of the cave, greenish yellow, with silver scales, and on its pointy backbone a young woman sat and waved.

"You're not a bad fellow," rumbled and grunted the dragon, and with every word, fire and sulfur rolled and the prince had to duck out of the way so as not to be singed. "Why do you want to fight me?"

"Because every year you come and take a maiden," the prince said staunchly. "And because you want to take my princess."

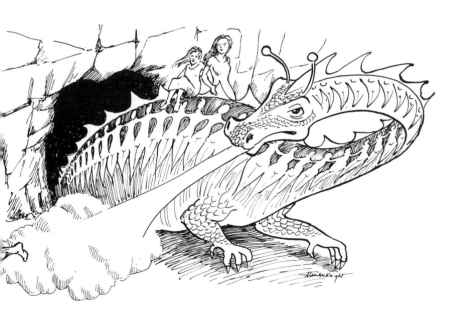

The woman on the back of the dragon began to giggle. The princess however stood on tiptoe and kissed the prince on his forehead. "Let's lose no time," she said.

He drew his sword, but stopped, perplexed, when he saw that with the help of the crone, she was climbing up on top of the dragon, grasping the hand of the smith's daughter, making herself comfortable on one of the silver scales.

The prince blinked his eyes, but quickly pulled himself together and plunged his sword courageously into the dragon's flank. The dragon only turned its head slightly and growled, "Get out of here!" He didn't have to say it twice, for the column of fire carried the young prince into the bushes, next to the sly servant, who picked him up, no longer seeing any more need to kill him. Then the dragon disappeared into the cave, never having shown its full length.

"I'm wounded," groaned the prince, and the two frustrated would-be lovers limped away together. As neither of the two had any desire to show up in front of the king, they set off on a journey.

In the meantime, the princess had passed through the cave on the back of the dragon. She was trembling with excitement and pressed up close against her friend. The cave soon opened up into a hidden meadow, which had big round boulders strewn about. On top of the boulders sat the women who had disappeared as maidens, waiting to welcome the princess.

There was a mighty greeting. The women were overjoyed, laughing and kissing each other. When they heard a shrill chirping, all took up the sound, whistling, trilling, hissing, and howling until from between the boulders, the dragon's grandmother stepped forth in a dress the color of the sea. She clapped her hands and the dragon spit a ring of fire in which all the women danced, and the princess knew that she was now a woman, too, for she bled like the others.

The celebration lasted the whole night. The dragon spit fireworks into the air. The animals of the woods joined them and danced, too. But slowly the women fell, one after another, into sleep. When it grew so still that even the dragon fell asleep, the dragon's grandmother went far beyond the boulders to a great black cauldron, under which a merry fire was burning.

In this cauldron, she cooked pictures and dreams. A delicious smell rose from it: some floated over the night-misted field out to the sea shore and blew over the sea; and some made its way out through the cave of the dragon into our world.

Sometimes even today a woman will sleep restlessly, and a great yearning will awaken in her for the cave of the dragon where the grandmother of us all cooks dreams.

My story is a lie, and like every lie, it contains some truth. And I know, you and I, we were there.

"The Princess Who Wouldn't Laugh"

In the old days, when the queens had lost their power and the kings wanted to decide everything, in the mountains there lived a king. He had become rich and mighty, for when his wife had died, he'd taken her land and, now and then, he waged wars to grow even richer and mightier. He had three daughters. According to law, the youngest was the heiress. His youngest daughter, however, was sick, very sick. She lived with her sisters in the tower of the castle. The castle was always cool and draughty. The sisters cuddled together under their furs and told each other stories.

But the older they became, the sadder they grew. For the king, to be honest, was really a horrid man. Anyone who didn't please him was quickly beheaded. The sisters feared him, but the youngest one feared him the most, for she knew that according to law she rightly would rule. Her father, however, wanted to keep everything and so he had to make her marry before her twenty-first birthday, when the power and possessions of her motherland reverted to her. He planned to marry her to a man who was on his side.

The more the youngest daughter pondered her fate, the sadder she became. Finally, she no longer wanted to eat and then, no longer laughed.

That didn't please the king at all. He couldn't possibly marry his daughter off with her so sick and pale. Already the people were muttering their suspicions that the king was secretly poisoning the crown princess.

The princess lay, shrouded in her furs, and stared at the wall. Her sisters tried in vain to cheer her up. They read her stories, put on plays for her, brought her delicate foods, but nothing helped. The princess, who was once so bloomingly pretty and merry, grew paler and sicker and thinner with each passing day.

The king was in despair. His conniving for power would be even more thwarted if his daughter died. So he had it proclaimed: "Whosoever can make my daughter laugh and eat again shall have her hand in marriage and half my kingdom as well."

With that he hoped to settle all of his problems with one blow. The princess, healthy and cheerful again, would rule half the kingdom with her husband and he would have the other half.

Many young men came: first the princes, then the dukes, then the knights, then the adventurers, and finally, occasionally, daring young peasants and shepherds took on the difficult task. But none of them succeeded in making the princess laugh, or even inspiring her to eat. Quite the contrary. With every failed effort, the princess grew thinner, more transparent. Finally, in his despair, the king had proclaimed: "Every young man who attempts to cure my daughter will be beheaded if he does not succeed."

The troops around the palace were reinforced. Doctors, healers, magicians, enchanters were called to the bed of the princess to save her life. But she sent them all away with a tired wave of her hand. Now hardly a man dared show himself at the palace. The severed heads (stuck on spears in front of the palace) of the few courageous ones who did try scared away further suitors.

The sisters kept the youngest princess apprised of the events. They were sad and worried and tried everything to cheer up their little sister. But with every new story, with every severed head, the little one grew more depressed and sad.

Finally no one else came. The king awaited the death of his youngest daughter. He began the preparations for the funeral march, chose wood for the coffin, bouquets and such. The sisters cried their eyes out and the mood in the palace was heavy.

Then one day, in the midst of the funeral preparations for the princess who hadn't even died yet, an old woman knocked on the castle gate. The sentry, nervous from the continual funeral preparations, overreacted, nearly throwing the crone over the edge of the drawbridge. She only giggled.

"It's surely a juggler," said the eldest and looked out the window. Then she shook her head and went back to the little sister's bed.

"Imagine that. It's a really old woman," she said.

With difficulty, the princess pulled herself up amidst her furs and pillows. "An old woman?" she asked in a weak voice. "I want to see her. Go to father and have the old woman called, please!"

She said that just in the nick of time, for the king was just advising the head sentry to chase the crone off . . . and if she wouldn't go of her own free will, to shove a spear through her old body. Why in God's name should he let the crone into the palace?

But now it was, so to speak, the last wish of his daughter, so he decided not to be overly particular and he had the crone fetched.

Like a dangerous criminal, she was led into the castle between two guards, taken through the castle courtyard, and over the plank to the tower. Instead of being afraid, she just looked around curiously and mumbled over and over to herself, "How can anyone be happy and healthy behind such cool walls. Unhealthy, damp, and decayed."

"Hold your mouth," the guard said nervously. The crone made him anxious. He felt uncomfortable walking beside her, but he didn't know why. Somehow she reminded him of his grandmother who had died a long time ago. She'd told him beautiful stories, but had forbidden him treats now and then, too. Under her sharp eyes he hadn't dared spear frogs and tear off their legs any more. She was from a world he didn't understand.

As if the crone had read his thoughts, she nodded to him in a friendly manner and looked deep into his eyes, into the wounds of his soul. Impatiently, he banged his spear against the stone wall.

Finally, they came to the door of the tower room. The sentries wanted
to come in with her, but the crone indicated with a motion of her hand
that they should stay standing there. As though under a spell, they
stopped and couldn't move an inch, although they were under orders
not to let the princess and the crone out of their sight.

After a while, they heard the deep voice of the old woman singing a
song.

> The soul is as old as a mountain.
> The soul is as deep as the sea.
> The soul is as wild as fire,
> And like a storm, the soul is free.
> Light as down, she flies up to heaven,
> Soft as water, slips under bedrock.
> And no one can catch her,
> No one can hold her.
> She always returns,
> And she always returns.

The high thin voice of the princess joined in the song of the crone,
". . . and she always returns."

And then the sentries heard the crone speak, but they couldn't understand what she was saying, for it sounded as though she said everything
backwards. As they listened, trying, the king came with his train of
attendants. He was about to throw a temper tantrum about the sentries
not following his orders, but as he stood in front of the door, the song
rose again, so magical and pure that tears appeared in his eyes. Secretly
everyone wiped their face, as the deep voice of the crone and the high
tender voice of the princess sang together.

As though nailed fast, the guard, the courtiers, and the king stood
before the door, all listening, not noticing that they couldn't move anymore.

In her room, the crone sat on the bed of the princess. To her right
and left were the two sisters, listening, lost in dreams. The crone had
taken the hand of the princess and looked into her eyes. She talked to
her in a foreign language and the princess smiled with tears running
down her face at the same time.

While the crone talked to her, the princess saw mountain cliffs, ocean
deeps, fairies at springs, wild women, dwarves, mosspeople. For the
crone was a woods-woman, an enchantress from ancient times, who
had fled with the last of her kin into the mountains, so they wouldn't
be murdered by the invading tribes of warriors. The princess listened
as the crone told of her life. She saw the huts of wood and straw that
the wild people had built in the shelter of the high cliffs. In her thoughts,
she accompanied the old woman through the woods, picked berries
and wild vegetables, and helped her bring wounded animals to her hut
to heal with herbs and juices. She watched how the old mountain

woman laid her hands on the wound and the edges slowly closed themselves. She saw a circle of elves at a spring and jumped with them through a waterfall. She gave them her hand and saw how, with glittering rainbows, the elves dissolved into mist.

Even deeper and happier she breathed, sighed, yawned, and stretched.

Finally the crone told of a warrior, feared all over. Attentively she followed the story of the war with the foreign tribes against the wild people, how the wild ones were pushed ever farther back into the mountains, and finally, how a defenseless group of peaceful people were driven together on a cliff to be slaughtered.

They were awaiting their death when a mountain woman came forth from their group and stepped up in front of the fabled warrior.

She raised her skirt, spread her legs and stepped forward. A ray of fire shot from her womb, while her mouth murmured phrases.

The legendary warrior started back. He'd never experienced anything like this. He began to back away. Then the wild woman let her skirt drop. She murmured an invocation and raised her arms. From her armpits streamed a smoke, a stink, a wind, that sent all the warriors reeling. Screaming and moaning they rolled and stumbled down the hill and fled.

At the last words of the crone, the princess giggled and laughed right heartily, repeating the funny part of the story again and again and bent double, almost rolling out of her bed with laughter. The crone laughed with her in a dark resonant voice, then showed the sisters how the mountain woman had lifted her skirts, had bared her armpits. The sisters had long since realized that the wild woman could only be this very same crone.

On the other side of the door all the faces wore astonished looks: the princess seemed to have laughed. They all listened even harder. Yes! A laugh! Happy sounds, giggles could be heard. The king beamed. In his mind he was already preparing to make the crone a wonderful reward. "Well, that's enough," he thought. "Now it's time for her to be on her way out."

But inside, things proceeded cheerfully with much giggling and storytelling. Then soft sighs and even moans. What was going on in the room? The men of the king looked at each other perplexed. But still they couldn't move. Long, long they stood there, while in the room of the princess a great party was going on.

An eternity seemed to pass until finally the door opened and the crone came out. She gave a pleasant wave of her hand and they could all move, stretch, bend yawn, cough. (Go pee!)

On her divan sat the princess and looked at all the men who were suddenly making an enormous noise. Then she had to laugh again and her sisters laughed right along with her.

The king didn't quite like the whole thing and wanted to get rid of the hag as soon as possible. Courtiers and sentries following, he hurried to the throne room, where he thought to reward her and send her on her way. He praised her high and low, with the appearance of much generosity, which only made the crone laugh slightly.

"We thank you," he said formally, "for having healed the princess. For indeed everyone in the palace can see that she's well. Take as a token of our thanks and acknowledgment this bag of gold."

His courtiers clapped and the king smiled benevolently as his servant handed her the bag, or rather, tried to hand her the bag, for the crone, in fact, had no intention of taking it.

"What do I want with your money?" she said craftily. "You promised half of your kingdom and the hand of the princess to the one who healed your daughter."

The courtiers looked at each other in astonishment.

The king let out a surprised grunt. "But you're a woman! How can I give you my daughter's hand? Take the gold and be satisfied before I change my mind."

Now the old woman wasn't at all surprised by this answer. She knew the powerful very well. When in need, they promise you the stars in the sky, but hardly have they been saved when they break every one of their promises, no longer believing them to be necessary.

"I want the hand of your daughter. I'll give you back the half of your kingdom," she said softly.

The king began to choke with rage. "You'll *give* me!" he croaked. He waved his arms around. "I'll have you imprisoned. I'll have you tortured. I'll have you thrown into the starvation tower. That'll teach you to be so shameless to a king."

"The king is the one who is shameless," the crone said with friendliness.

The courtiers howled in outrage. That she should dare!

"You're dealing with a very old and powerful queen," the old woman said softly. "But that's not so important. You've given your promise and now wish to break it. That weighs very heavily, king. Think carefully."

The king was about ready to begin hollering, when the gaze of the crone met his. He wasn't stupid, and he recognized at once that she was not only his born equal but, in fact, his superior.

She grew before his eyes. Became wide and tall and stately. She wore a dress which was both the color of the shimmering sea and the ice gray of mountain rock. Her hair shone dark and mysterious.

He couldn't take his eyes off the woman who had transformed herself in such an amazing way. Yes, he began to desire her. He groped under her ever-changing dress for her breasts, her belly. He breathed heavily, he stretched his arms out to her and swayed. He felt sick with longing. Tears ran from his eyes. He didn't understand what was happening to him.

"What . . . is . . . it . . .?" he muttered and fell into the arms of his men. "I'm blind, I can't see anymore."

Excited murmurs and coughs ran through the hall. The old crone waved her hand softly and smiled.

"King," she said gently, "think it over well before you tell me your final decision. And know that your word does not weigh as heavily with me as the wish of the princess. And she wants to go with me."

Released from his spell, the king howled, "You, you shabby old crow! You witch! You!! Capture her!" he screamed in the shrillest of tones. "Bind her and throw her in the tower, quarter her."

The sentries stumbled around. But the old woman disappeared before their eyes.

Reinforcements were added to the sentries at the castle gate. No one would volunteer to guard, so they had to be assigned in shifts. And at that, they would only do their duty under threat of severe punishment. Gossip was making the rounds about the old witch: she could bewitch, castrate, kill. The guardsmen's swords were small comfort to them, as they huddled in the cold in front of the gate.

The king was moody and unpredictable. He screamed at his courtiers, cursed and threatened them. Each morning he woke up hating himself for having dreamed of the crone, the crone who had transformed herself so wonderfully in front of his eyes.

Only in the tower of the princess was anyone happy. All three sisters zealously sewed fur coats (much to the disapproval of their ladies) and knitted thick wool socks. They told each other stories the whole day long, and laughed and sang the song of the old woman again and again, the youngest singing the melody and the two sisters finding beautiful harmonies to go with it. Even the stiff court ladies leaned back and listened to the song.

Something was in the air. Everyone could feel it. But no one could name it.

The princesses were peaceful and happy. The general moodiness, anxiety and confusion only gave them further reason to be merry.

One day, just as the king had returned from a foray, and all his men and horses were gathered in the courtyard, he heard excited screams.

As the king hurried towards where the screaming was the loudest, he saw how the people were pointing into the air with their fingers. He raised his face to the sky and couldn't believe what he saw: flying above was a gigantic eagle, carrying a person on its back. Fascinated, the king watched the flight of the eagle, then he froze. On the back of the bird sat the crone. She waved at him, and he could even hear her deep laughter.

The eagle steered straight for the tower of the princess. The king ran from the castle courtyard into the open and looked up to the outer window of the tower. Never for a moment did it occur to him to try and stop what was going on. He stared at the eagle as though under a spell. The bird flew to the window of the youngest princess.

Briefly, the king covered his eyes as the princess, wrapped in a thick fur coat and socks, stepped out of the window and swung herself up to the crone on the back of the eagle. When he looked again that eagle had grasped a bundle of furs in which the two elder sisters sat.

The princesses waved to the king and his courtiers and away flew the eagle with the mountain woman, the princess, and her sisters.

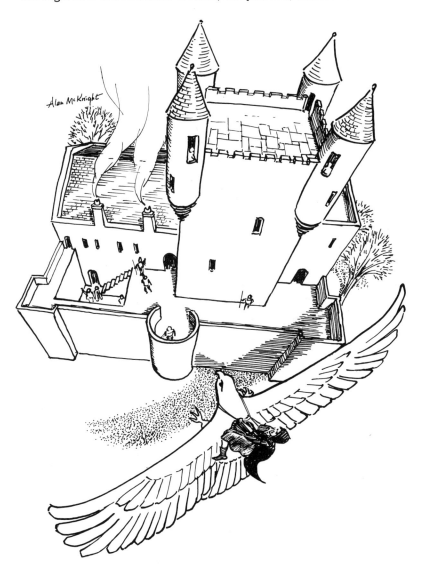

The king sank to the ground and died of fright on the spot. The castle began to fall apart. Peasants and shepherds broke up the stone walls and took the stones to build themselves houses and huts.

Still, on clear moonlit nights, the inhabitants of the mountain villages run to their front doors to listen. They can hear the old mountain woman laughing and singing with the princesses. The wind carries back a piece of their song through the night:

> No one can catch her
> No one can hold her
> Instead she returns
>   She
>   Always
>   Returns.

Dragontime Resources

Women's Blood Mysteries Workshops available through:

Brooke Medicine Eagle, PO Box 1682, Helena, MT 59624

Mary Greer, 15321 Wet Hill Rd., Nevada City, CA 95959

Carol McGrath, 3730 Press Ave., Victoria, BC, Canada V8X 2Z1

Jean Mountaingrove, Sunny Valley, OR 97497

Christina Nealson and Carole Shane, 3305 4th St., Boulder, CO 80304

Vicki Noble, PO Box 5544, Berkeley, CA 94705

Barbara Smith, 1515 Fell St., Victoria, BC, Canada V8R 1P5

Spider, 111 Branch St., Pittsburgh, PA 15215

Susun Weed, PO Box 64DT, Woodstock, NY 12498

For Dragon Maidens
Those Who Await the Bleeding

The Clear Red Stone: A Myth and the Meaning of Menstruation, Alexandra Kolkmeyer, 1982, In Sight, 535 Cordova Rd. #228, Santa Fe, NM 87501

Flowering Woman: Moontime for Kory, Mary Dillon with Shinan Barclay, 1988, Sunlight, PO Box 1300, Sedona, AZ 86336

PERIOD. JoAnn Loulan, Bonnie Lopez, Marcia Quackenbush, Volcano, PO Box 270, Volcano, CA 95689

Red Flower: Rethinking Menstruation, Dena Taylor, 1988, Crossing Press, Freedom, CA 95019

For Dragon Mothers
Those Who Bleed and Do Not Die

"Lifting the Curse of Menstruation," *Women & Health*, Vol. 8, No. 2/3, Fall 1983, Haworth Press, 28 East 22 St., NYC, NY 10010

Lunar Phase Calendar, Snake and Snake, Rt. 3, Box 165, Durham, NC 27713 (The best menstrual/lunar chart! And it's only a dollar.)

Menstrual Goddesses from Cindy Leespring, 816½ Cm. Sierra Vista, Santa Fe, NM 87501

A Menstrual Journey, poetry by Judith Barr, PO Box 552, Pound Ridge, NY 10576

Moon Diary and Love Charms, Elizabeth Pepper, Pentacle, PO Box 348, Cambridge, MA 02238

Moon Time and *Moon Lodge,* Brook Medicine Eagle, Harmony Network, PO Box 2550, Guerneville, CA, 95446

Self-Ritual for Invoking Release of Spirit Life in the Womb, Deborah Maia, Mother Spirit Publishing, PO Box 893, Great Barrington, MA 01230

For Dragon Crones
Those Who Keep Their Wise Blood Inside

Book About Menopause, Montreal Health Press, PO Box 1000, Station Place du Parc, Montreal, Quebec, Canada, H2W 2N1

The Crone: Woman of Age, Wisdom, & Power, Barbara Walker, 1985, Harper & Row

The Gift of Menopause, RAJ, PO Box 18599, Denver, CO 80218

Menopause Self-Care Manual, Santa Fe Health Education Project, PO Box 577, Santa Fe, NM 87504

For Dragontimes
Periodicals . . .

Sage Woman, PO Box 5130, Santa Cruz, CA 95063 (single copy $6)

Snake Power, 5856 College Ave., #138, Oakland, CA 94618 ($6.50)

Woman of Power, PO Box 827, Cambridge, MA 02238 ($6)

Womanspirit, 1974-1984, still available from Box 263, Wolf Creek, OR 97497

Altar pieces . . .

Ancient Art, PO Box 7485, Santa Cruz, CA 95061

Chocolate Goddesses, Lyricon, 83½ Partition St., Saugerties, NY 12477; (914) 246-7992

Gaia Catalog Company, 1442-A Walnut St. #184, N. Berkeley, CA 94709

Goddesses by Joann Colbert, 4141 Ball Rd. #178, Cypress, CA 90630

Goddess Images by Jay Goldspinner, 61 Stafford St., Worcester, MA 01603

Halcyon Arts, PO Box 7153, Halcyon, CA 93420

In Her Image, 816½ Cm. Sierra Vista, Santa Fe, NM 87501

Jane Iris Designs, PO Box 608, Graton, CA 95444

Matrika Birthing Amulet, from Lynn Marsh, 804 Bryant St., Palo Alto, CA 94301

Ravenwood, PO Box 1035, Easthampton, MA 01027

Star River Productions, PO Box 6254, N. Brunswick, NJ 08902

Suppressed Histories Archives, Max Dashu PO Box 3511, Oakland, CA 94609

Ways of Our Grandmothers, 215 Hames Rd., Corralitos, CA 95076

Dragons . . .

Dragon Shirt for kids, folks, and big women:
Snake and Snake, Rt. 3, Box 165, Durham, NC 27713

Everything in dragons:
Dancing Dragons, 1881 Fieldbrook Rd., Arcata, CA 95521
(800) 322-6040

Essential oils and . . .

Aromalamp, 369 Montezuma, Suite 111, Santa Fe, NM 87501; (800) 933-5267

Aromatherapy for Women, Maggie Tisserand, Healing Arts, 1985

Essential Oil Co., PO Box 88, Sandy, OR, 97055; (503) 695-2400

Audio tapes . . .

A Circle is Cast, Libana, PO Box 530, Cambridge, MA 02140

Cauldron Journey for Healing, by Nicki Scully with Jerry Garcia, PO Box 5025, Eugene, OR 97405

Delphys: Sacred Spaces for Inner Journeys, Amy Fradon, Cathie Malach, Leslie Ritter, Kim Rosen, PO Box 174, Bearsville, NY 12409

Goddess Suite and Stories, Cynthia Crossen and Louise Kessel, Rt. 2, Box 435, Pittsboro, NC 27312

Invocation to Free Women, Circle of Aradia, 4111 Lincoln Blvd. #211, Marina del Rey, CA 90292

Moon Time and *Moon Lodge,* Brook Medicine Eagle, Harmony Network, PO Box 2550, Guerneville, CA, 95446

Opening the Heart of the Womb, Ondrea and Steven Levine, 4 Cielo Ln. #4, Novato, CA 94949

Songs for the Seasons, Aradia, Mary Ann Fusco, 720 S. 44th St., Boulder, CO 80303

Songs of the Spirit, Prayers for the Planet, and *Songs of Transformation,* Lisa Thiel, 821 West Utopia Rd., Phoenix AZ 85027

We All Come From the Goddess, Tori Rea, Molly Scott, Sarah Benson, Medicine Song, 156 Sullivan St. #19, NYC, NY 10012

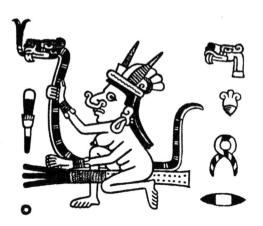

Tlazolteotl, Aztec goddess of witchcraft, rides on a serpent, the symbol of sexuality. Her broom is intended to sweep away the sins of mankind.

Dragontime References

Arachne, *Journal of Matriarchal Studies*, London, 1986

Shinan Naom Barclay, *Moontime Anthology: A Call to Power, A Return to the Sacred*, Sunlight, 1990

B. Bettelheim, *Symbolic Wounds: Puberty Rites and the Envious Male*, Glencoe, IL, 1954

Judy Chicago,
  The Dinner Party, New York, 1979
  The Birth Project, Doubleday, 1985

Barbara Christian and R. Snowden, *Patterns and Perceptions of Menstruation: A World Health Orginization study in Egypt, India, Indonesia, Jamaica, Mexico, Pakistan, Philippines, Korea, England, and Yugoslavia*, St. Martin's, 1983

Emily Culpepper, "The Muse As Medusa," *Woman of Power*, Winter/Spring 1986

Mary Daly, *Gyn/Ecology: The Metaethics of Radical Feminism*, Beacon, 1978

Katharina Dalton, *Once a Month*, Hunter House, 1979

Alice Dan with Carol Leppa, "The Menstrual Cycle Research," *Women's Health Perspectives*, Vol 1, Oryx, 1988

H. Debrunner, *Witchcraft in Ghana*, Accra, 1961

Janice Delaney, Mary Jane Lupton, and Emily Toth, *The Curse: A Cultural History of Menstruation*, revised, U of Illinois Press, 1988

G. Devereux, *Baubo. Die mythische Vulva*, Frankfurt, 1981

E. M. Dewan, "On the possibility of a perfect rhythm method of birth control by periodic light stimulation," *Amer. Journal of Obstetrics and Gynecology* 99:1016-1019, 1967

P. Dickinson, *Das grosse Buch der Drachen*, Oldenburg, 1981

Mary Dillon with Shinan Barclay, *Flowering Woman: Moontime for Kory,* Sunlight, 1987

Susan and N. Drury, *Healing Oils and Essences,* Harper & Row (Australia), 1987

L. Durdin-Robertson, *The Goddesses of Chaldea, Syria, and Egypt,* Clonegal, 1975

Mircea Eliade,
Patterns in Comparative Religion, New York, 1958
Encyclopedia of Religion, Macmillan, 1987

Federation of Feminist Women's Health Centers,
How To Stay Out of the Gynecologist's Office, 1981
A New View of a Woman's Body, 1981

J. G. Frazer, *The Golden Bough: A Study in Magic and Religion,* London, 1890, then Macmillan (abridged), 1963

Luisa Francia,
Mond, Tanz, Magie, FrauenOffensive, Munich, 1983
Hexen Tarot (Witches' Tarot), Munich, 1985
Der Afrikanische Traum, Zurich, 1985

Le Goff, "Saint Marcellus of Paris and the Dragon," in *Time, Work and Culture in the Middle Ages,* Chicago, 1980

Marija Gimbutas,
The Goddesses and Gods of Old Europe, U of California Press, 1982
The Language of the Goddess, Harper & Row, 1989

Naomi Goldenberg, *Changing of the Gods,* Beacon Press, 1979

Grimm, *The Complete Fairy Tales of the Brothers Grimm,* Bantam, 1812, 1857, 1987

Sadja Greenwood, *Menopause, Naturally,* Volcano, 1984

Rumer Godden, *The Dragon of Og,* Viking, 1981

H. G. Gorer, *Africa Dances,* New York, 1935

Alma Gottlieb & T. Buckley, *Blood Magic: The Anthropology of Menstruation,* U of California Press, 1988

R. Graves, *The White Goddess,* Noonday, 1988

Esther Harding, *Woman's Mysteries,* Harper Colophon, 1971

Heresies Great Goddess Issue, New York, 1982

P. Hogarth with Val Clery, *Dragons,* Jonathan-James, Viking Toronto, 1979

Keri Hulme, *The Bone People,* New Zealand/London, 1986

E. Ingersoll, *Dragons and Dragon Lore,* Payson & Clarke, New York, 1928

Kris Jeter, "Cinderella: Her Multi-Layered Puissant Messages Over Millennia," in *Marriage and Family Review*, Vol.7, No.4, Winter 1984, Haworth

Shirley Johnson and L. F. Snow, "Modern-day Menstrual Folklore: Some Clinical Implications," *Journal of the American Medical Association*, No. 25, June 1977

Catherine Keller, *From A Broken Web*, Beacon, 1986

Helen King, "Born to Bleed: Artemis and Greek Women," in *Images of Women in Antiquity*, Wayne State U Press, 1983

Leslie Kotin, *The Feminine Moebius: Understanding the Menstrual Cycle*, 1985

C. Kluckhohn, *Navaho Witchcraft*, Boston, 1967

Alexandra Kolkmeyer, *The Clear Red Stone: A Myth and the Meaning of Menstruation*, InSight, 1983

Lady-Unique-Inclination of the Night, No. 1-5, New Brunswick, 1976-81

Louise Lander, *Images of Bleeding: Menstruation as Ideology*, Orlando, 1988

"Lifting the Curse of Menstruation: A Feminist Appraisal of the Influence of Menstruation on Women's Lives," *Women & Health*, Vol. 8, No. 2/3, Fall 1983, Haworth Press

Hanny Lightfoot-Klein, *Prisoners of Ritual: An Odyssey into Female Genital Circumcision in Africa*, Harrington Park, 1989

Lucy Lippsard, *Overlay*, New York, 1983

JoAnn Gardner-Loulan, Bonnie Lopez, Marcia Quackenbush, *PERIOD*, Volcano, 1981

Ann Mankowitz, *Change of Life: A Psychological Study of Dreams and Menopause*, Inner City, 1984

Patricia Monaghan, *The Book of Goddesses and Heroines*, Llewellyn, 1990

Margaret Murray, *The Witch Cult in Western Europe*, New York, 1971

P. Newman, *The Hill of the Dragon*, Bath, 1979

Rina Nissim, *Natural Healing in Gynecology*, Pandora, 1986

Vicki Noble, *Female Blood, Roots of Shamanism*, Shaman's Drum, Spring 1986

E. Novak, MD, *The Superstition and Folklore of Menstruation*, John Hopkins Hospital Bulletin 27, September 1916

Wendy D. O'Flaherty, *Women, Androgynes, and Other Mythical Beasts*, U of Chicago Press, 1980

Jane Porcino, *Growing Older, Getting Better,* Addison-Wesley, 1983

Rosetta Reitz, *Menopause, A Positive Approach,* Penguin, 1979

E. H. Schafer, *The Divine Woman: Dragon Ladies and Rain Maidens in T'ang literature,* U of California Press, 1973

Penelope Shuttle and P. Redgrave, *The Wise Wound: Menstruation,* Bantam, 1990

Merlin Stone,
   Ancient Mirrors of Womanhood, Beacon, 1979
   When God Was A Woman, HBJ/Harvest, 1976

Dena Taylor, *Red Flower: Rethinking Menstruation,* Crossing, 1988

Ann Voda, Myra Dinnerstein, and Sheryl O'Donnell, *Changing Perspectives on Menopause,* U of Texas Press, 1982

Barbara Walker,
   The Crone, Harper & Row, 1985
   Woman's Dictionary of Symbols and Sacred Objects, Harper & Row, 1988
   Woman's Encyclopedia of Myths and Secrets, Harper & Row, 1983

Susun Weed,
   Wise Woman Herbal for the Childbearing Year, Ash Tree, 1986
   Healing Wise; The Second Wise Woman Herbal, Ash Tree, 1989

Paula Weideger, *Menstruation & Menopause: The Physiology and Psychology, the Myth and the Reality,* Delta, 1977

Jennifer and R. J. Woolger, *The Goddess Within*, Fawcett Columbine, 1989

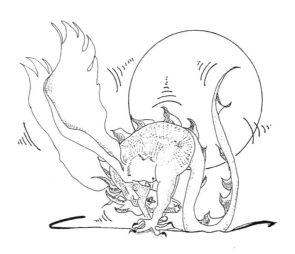

Index

Susun Weed, born 1946 in Ohio, loves women, witches, weeds, writing, drawing, and organizing. Ash Tree Publishing is the material result of the convergence of these loves. She is joined in this work by her daughter, Justine Swede, who's on her way to becoming a renowned chef. (The cover dragon was drawn for Justine in 1973 as a protector figure.)

In addition to publishing, Susun tends goats, creates rituals, teaches herbal medicine, gardens, and cooks. She is the founder of the Wise Woman Center: safe space for women learning and healing. Susun is working on a series of ten Wise Woman Herbals, the first two of which, *For the Childbearing Year* (1986) and *Healing Wise* (1989), are already cherished classics of simple, safe, self-care suggestions.

"Editing *Dragontime* was involving, intense and passionate yet meandering, unpredictable, and dramatic—altogether encompassing, just like moon time. As I edited and re-edited Sasha's translation of Luisa's work, across the ocean, Luisa was translating my words into German for *Heilweise (Healing Wise)*. Such a marvelous, luscious tangle of tongues! My notes are in brackets [like this] in the text. I've a feeling this book will go to press at the dark of the moon, at dragontime."

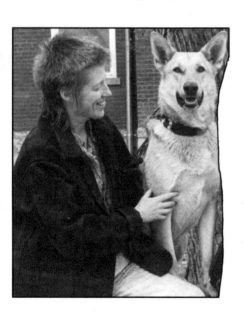

Mau Blossom, artist and midwife, found inspiration for *Zabu* the dragon in the woods of her Ozark mountain farm. "Chinese doctors study art along with their other courses on the human body—they believe it puts them in touch with the creative, healing parts of the mind. I agree. I'm primarily a midwife and woman's health care practitioner, but I'm also very involved with woman and nature-inspired art. My cartoon strip "Amaz-Egret" is serialized in a feminist paper, and other work is regularly seen in feminist and environmental publications, often under the by-line *Daucus-Blossom*."

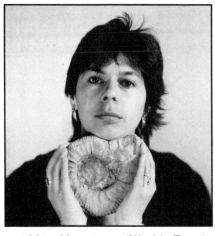

Luisa Francia, born in Germany, is a well-loved and well-respected author, screenwriter, and ritualist. Her works include a daughter, born 1974, seven screenplays and TV film scripts including "Hexen" (Witches) and "Das zweite Erwachen der Christa Klages" (The Second Awakening of Christa Klages), and six books:

1981: *Hexentarot (Witch's Tarot)*

1982: *Berühre Wega, kehr zur Erde zurück (Touch Vega, Return to Earth*, feminist astrology.

1984: *Kalypso (Calypso)*, initiations into women's mysteries, trances, dreams, visions.

1985: *Der afrikanische Traum (The African Dream)*, diaries of her work with a West African fetish-priestess.

1986: *Mond Tanz Magie (Moon Dance Magic)*, the lunar, thirteen-month year highlights thirteen mythic women, thirteen aspects of woman spirit/woman power, and thirteen moon dance rituals.

1988: *Drachenzeit (Dragontime)*, the magic and mystery of menstruation from fairy tale to every-day and into what-if.

1989: *Zaubergarn (Tangle of Yarns)*, magical stories of ordinary things.

Luisa's home is filled with goddesses, hundreds of goddesses, goddesses of every size and incredible shapes. She follows the Wise Woman Ways.

Want more of Luisa in English? Send us a postcard with your top two choices for the next translation.

Sasha Daucus, born 1959 in Oakland, California, is a feminist writer and translator whose main interest is women's emotional and physical health. Before settling down in Missouri, she spent time outside the country, including study on a scholarship from the University of Bonn, West Germany. "Translating is like traveling: you connect with people who are different from you through your similarities and get a chance to see yourself better because of your differences."

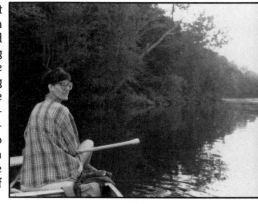

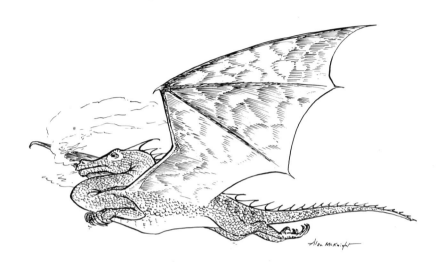

Best Sellers
by Susun Weed
from
Ash Tree Publishing

Wise Woman Herbal for the Childbearing Year
40,000 copies in print

"Don't let the title fool you—this book contains valuable information for everyone and is in constant use in our house."

Herbal treatments for common difficulties before, during, and after pregnancy including herbs for birth control and herbs for infant care.

"Coupled with sound dietary pointers and how-to hints, Susun's herbal advice for pregnant women—and their helpers—is indispensable."

Healing Wise:
The Second Wise Woman Herbal

"Far more than an herbal reference, this book is infused with spiritual, mystical, historical, as well as personal references for natural healing."

"A magnificent contribution to the progressive thought related to healing and how it actually occurs in the body. A book for anyone on a journey to wholeness."

"Plant talk, herbal recipes, weed walks, fairies at play, and solid information make this my favorite herbal. Even teaches your kids!"

Available in bookstores or order directly.

Please send _____ copies of *Childbearing Year* at $8.95.
Please send _____ copies of *Healing Wise* at $11.95.
Include $3 shipping per order. New York State residents please add tax.

Name _____

Address _____

_____

Make checks payable to Ash Tree Publishing. U.S. funds only.